Counselor's Resource
on
Psychiatric Medications

COUNSELOR'S RESOURCE
ON
PSYCHIATRIC MEDICATIONS

ISSUES OF TREATMENT AND REFERRAL

GEORGE BUELOW
University of Southern Mississippi

SUZANNE HEBERT

Brooks/Cole Publishing Company

I(T)P™ An International Thomson Publishing Company

Pacific Grove • Albany • Bonn • Boston • Cincinnati • Detroit • London • Madrid • Melbourne
Mexico City • New York • Paris • San Francisco • Singapore • Tokyo • Toronto • Washington

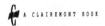
A CLAIREMONT BOOK

Sponsoring Editor: *Claire Verduin*
Editorial Associate: *Gay C. Bond*
Production Editor: *Laurel Jackson*
Production Assistant: *Tessa A. McGlasson*
Manuscript Editor: *Kay Mikel*

Permissions Editor: *Cathleen S. Collins*
Interior and Cover Design: *Laurie Albrecht*
Indexer: *James Minkin*
Typesetting: *Joan Mueller Cochrane*
Printing and Binding: *Malloy Lithographing, Inc.*

For more information, contact:

BROOKS/COLE PUBLISHING COMPANY
511 Forest Lodge Road
Pacific Grove, CA 93950
USA

International Thomson Publishing Europe
Berkshire House 168–173
High Holborn
London WC1V 7AA
England

Thomas Nelson Australia
102 Dodds Street
South Melbourne, 3205
Victoria, Australia

Nelson Canada
1120 Birchmont Road
Scarborough, Ontario
Canada M1K 5G4

International Thomson Editores
Campos Eliseos 385, Piso 7
Col. Polanco
11560 México D. F. México

International Thomson Publishing GmbH
Königswinterer Strasse 418
53227 Bonn
Germany

International Thomson Publishing Asia
221 Henderson Road
#05–10 Henderson Building
Singapore 0315

International Thomson Publishing Japan
Hirakawacho Kyowa Building, 3F
2-2-1 Hirakawacho
Chiyoda-ku, Tokyo 102
Japan

Printed in the United States of America

10   9   8   7   6   5   4   3   2   1

THIS BOOK IS PRINTED ON ACID-FREE RECYCLED PAPER

Library of Congress Cataloging-in-Publication Data
Buelow, George, [date]
    Counselor's resource on psychiatric medications : issues of treatment and referral / George Buelow, Suzanne Hebert.
        p.   cm.
    Includes bibliographical references and index.
    ISBN 0-534-24960-4
    1. Mental illness—Chemotherapy. 2. Psychotropic drugs.
3. Psychopharmacology. 4. Chronic pain—Chemotherapy. I. Hebert,
Suzanne, [date]. II. Title.
    [DNLM: 1. Mental Disorders—drug therapy. 2. Psychotropic Drugs—therapeutic use. 3. Pain—drug therapy.   WM 402 B928c 1995]
RC483.B84 1995
616.89'18--dc20
DNLM/DLC
for Library of Congress   94-16311
                                                                    CIP

CONTENTS

PREFACE

This book is an introduction for counselors to the treatment and referral issues that surround commonly prescribed psychiatric drugs. It provides an overview of psychopharmacology as it affects counselors' work with clients who are already using psychiatric medications or who potentially should be. This book provides up-to-date information on the mechanisms of action and side effects of typically prescribed psychiatric medications, including antidepressants, antianxiety agents, antipsychotics, and pain medications.

Because of the recent explosion of knowledge through biochemistry research, psychopharmacology texts have become difficult for many counselors to read and fully understand. Even so, counselors often work with clients who are taking psychiatric medications with which neither client nor counselor are familiar. Not only are counselors faced with a wide range of medications, but they also are often at a loss about how to work with prescribing physicians. In addition, many counselors do not know whether or how to work on medical compliance issues as central concerns in therapy. Contemporary jobs in counseling, both in private and public practice, require a clear understanding of pharmacopsychological issues. We define pharmacopsychological issues as those within the scope of practice of psychologists who are being trained to prescribe psychiatric drugs.

We wrote this book as (a) an introductory text for those studying drugs used in treating mental illness; (b) a reference for advanced undergraduate and graduate students in counseling, guidance, nursing, social work, and psychology; and (c) a resource for counselors and practitioners who work in the field and often have only the *Physicians' Desk Reference* (PDR) as a guide to understanding the psychiatric drugs used by their clients. In *Counselor's Resource on Psychiatric Medications*, each chapter is meant to stand alone so that, without having to review other chapters, readers can refer to a particular diagnostic area, the drugs most frequently used, their usual actions, and their side effects.

This book is organized under headings that are familiar to clinicians. It begins with an introductory chapter in which we examine treatment and referral issues that counselors face when working with clients. The next chapter contains information about the components of neurophysiology and neurotransmission. Then, in Chapters 2 through 5, we discuss the major psychiatric disorders for which clients are most likely to be using psychiatric drugs: depression and manic depression, anxiety and panic disorders, psychosis, and pain. (We included the chapter on pain because chronic pain usually has both a physical and psychogenic side and because pain medications often produce psychiatric effects.)

Chapters 2 through 5 each begin with an introduction to the etiology of a specific psychiatric problem, followed by a discussion of the mechanisms of action for the classes of drugs used to treat the problem, so that counselors can better understand the medical intention of the drugs. In these chapters, we discuss the most common drug treatments, drug and therapy interaction, and referral issues that arise within a specific diagnostic area. Throughout this book, we emphasize the need for an understanding of how various drugs influence the workings of the nervous system through neurotransmission and, thus, the symptomatology of the psychiatric disorder.

To assist readers further, we have included two appendices in this book, as well as a glossary. The first appendix is an overview of the components that make up the central nervous system. The second is a discussion of pharmacokinetics— the study of in vivo drug processes, including administration, absorption, distribution, metabolism, and excretion.

ACKNOWLEDGMENTS

We wish to acknowledge the people whose support, encouragement, and suggestions have helped us in writing this book. First, we want to thank those who reviewed earlier versions of the manuscript, including Thomas McGovern, Texas Tech Health Sciences Center; Dorothy Neufeld, Loma Linda University; and Howard J. Shaffer, Harvard Medical School–The Cambridge Hospital.

Further, we want to thank our colleagues in the Psychology Department at the University of Southern Mississippi for their support—especially John Alcorn, Chairman; Lillian Range; Mark Leach; and Mike Chavetz.

We would also like to thank the staff at Brooks/Cole, especially Claire Verduin, Laurie Albrecht, Gay C. Bond, Cat Collins, Laurel Jackson, Tessa McGlasson, and E. Kelly Shoemaker, as well as manuscript editor Kay Mikel, for their assistance in developing and publishing this book.

George Buelow
Suzanne Hebert

Counseling and Psychiatric Medicines

Referral of clients to psychiatrists or to nonpsychiatrist family physicians for appraisal has a strong emotional and ethical push or pull for many counselors. When asked if they would feel comfortable making referrals for psychiatric drug intervention, a significant minority of graduate counseling students in our classes respond that they don't believe people should use drugs for emotional problems, especially for anxiety and depression. As the issue is debated in class, salient features of counselors' beliefs about drugs, usually in the absence of course work in pharmacopsychology, are that (a) drugs should be a last resort and should be used primarily to treat psychoses (schizophrenia, for example); (b) psychiatric drugs do not differ a great deal from recreational drugs people use to relieve boredom or depression (cocaine, for example) or anxiety (alcohol and narcotics, for example); (c) such a wide gulf exists between counselors and psychiatrists that communication is difficult or impossible; (d) learning about psychiatric drugs is difficult and working with clients who are on psychiatric drugs, or referring them, will raise counselors' malpractice liability; and (e) drugs cannot cure mental illnesses and, thus, are not superior to psychotherapy or even to a placebo. Unfortunately, this belief system, which comes less from experience than from family and societal values, is often shared by the counselors and the clients they see.

Due to the lack of emphasis on biopsychological training in counseling programs, many counselors and counseling psychologists are not prepared in

pharmacopsychology. The belief systems of counselors often inhibit them from gaining practical experience in this important area. This is reinforced by the limited educational opportunities available that could provide insight and encourage practical experience. This lack of preparation has slowed the development of the counseling field in two ways. At the individual level, it has hindered counselors' effectiveness in working with clients who are taking psychiatric drugs and has impeded referral of clients who need both psychiatric medications and psychotherapy. And, at the professional level, counselors' lack of expertise in this rapidly developing area reflects on the stature of counseling as a force within the competitive community of health care providers. This lack of expertise also presents ethical problems. Is it ethical to work with clients using traditional counseling techniques alone when a great deal of suffering could be alleviated, and the counseling process could itself be enhanced, by judicious use of psychiatric medications?

Finally, legal problems may well emerge if counselors are not both informed and prudent in their decisions to treat and refer clients who are in need of psychiatric medications. The liability incurred in not referring a client for appraisal who needs psychiatric medication is certainly much higher than that of referring a client who does not. Good faith referral of clients is the responsibility of counselors; the decision to prescribe rests with the psychiatrist or the nonpsychiatrist physician.

Today, counselors are trained to work with an increasingly more difficult client population. In community mental health centers, college counseling centers, and private practice, counselors face a variety of difficult and complex psychiatric cases. National certification requires that counselors and counseling psychologists be trained to provide expertise in developmental deficiencies, crisis intervention, remediation of emotional problems, couples and family therapy, accurate appraisal and assessment, and consultation within the community. Psychiatric medications may be in use in any one of these areas. For example, counselors assess and work with children who have been diagnosed as having attention deficit disorder with hyperactivity. Many of these children may have been taking methylphenidate (Ritalin) for various periods of time. Individuals in crisis, whom counselors commonly see, have often been prescribed tranquilizers or sedative hypnotic agents without adequate psychological assessment. Finally, even if certification and licensure for psychotherapists and psychologists did not support development of expertise in these areas, the pragmatics of both public and private practice certainly would. Knowledge of the use of psychiatric medications is clearly becoming a necessary step in the development of the science and art of counseling.

This book is designed to provide up-to-date information on what counselors have traditionally been expected to know, such as referral to psychiatric physicians and support for drug compliance. However, it also provides a firm base in areas that counselors are increasingly confronting, such as the **neuropharmacology** of typically prescribed psychiatric medications. Regardless of where you stand on the issues, future counseling and clinical psychologists, as psychiatric health care providers with hospital privileges, may well be expected to know psychiatric medications well enough to prescribe them! These **pharmacopsychologists** are already being trained in national and state-sponsored postdoctoral programs.

TREATMENT ISSUES

Counselors are routinely faced with a number of converging problems with clients' use of psychiatric medications. First, counselors are expected to understand the experience and side-effect problems clients have with their medications. Second, counselors are expected to know the conditions under which clients should be referred to a physician for appraisal for medication. Third, counselors are expected to help clients with drug compliance. Fourth, expectations are rising that psychotherapists should be able to educate clients about the interactions of their psychiatric medications and alcohol or illicit drugs and to understand issues of dual diagnosis. A useful understanding of each of these areas presupposes a general knowledge of pharmacopsychology, including neurotransmitters and drug interactions as well as specific knowledge of frequently prescribed antidepressant, antianxiety, and antipsychotic medications.

REFERRAL ISSUES

Perhaps as challenging as working with clients on medication issues, counselors must learn to talk effectively with physicians about the efficacy, side effects, and compliance problems that may stem from each client's medications. Counselors also must establish good working relationships with physicians in the local psychiatric community so they can effectively refer their clients when necessary. The referral picture is complicated by the fact that most antianxiety and antidepressant drugs (around 70 percent) are prescribed by family and other physicians not extensively trained in psychiatry.

Two of the most frequently prescribed medications, benzodiazepines (antianxiety agents such as Valium) and fluoxetine (Prozac for depression), are usually not lethal in suicide attempts when taken in moderate doses or alone (without other drugs to potentiate them). Thus, family physicians feel, perhaps unwisely, at lower risk in prescribing them. Further, because psychiatrists' office charges are often more expensive than a visit to a family physician, patients quite reasonably are more likely to choose the latter. Finally, because for many people there is an onus on visiting a psychiatrist, patients are more likely to go to their family physician initially for depression or anxiety.

Many physicians are not as aware of the benefits of psychotherapy for their patients as they might be. Although the picture is changing rapidly, many physicians still do not commonly refer patients for counseling services in the community or utilize feedback from mental health workers as effectively as they might. It is, therefore, the responsibility of counselors to open contact with psychiatrist and nonpsychiatrist physicians in their communities to begin a dialogue about patient medications.

Even though counselors should not be responsible for med-checks, physicians need as much independent feedback on the patient's social adaptation and medication compliance as possible. To provide this information on request to a physician or to initiate contact, counselors must remember to have clients provide written consent. Like psychologists, physicians want and need feedback that is accurate, specific, and timely. It is best, therefore, to have the most salient issues written down and the chart available before contacting a client's physician by phone. Phone contacts should be followed up in writing so specifics of the conversation are reflected in the written record. If clear liaisons are built in a personal way, many physicians are willing to see clients to evaluate them for possible psychiatric medication on the recommendation and referral of counselors and other psychotherapists.

When making referrals for drug screening, even in cases where the client has chosen his or her family physician, it is important to first obtain a written consent from the client to contact and to forward records to the nurse case managers and to the physician. At that time, a letter should be sent to the physician outlining the behavioral, observational cues that occasioned the referral. Psychological judgments and interpretations should be kept to a minimum, and psychological jargon should not be used. As a general rule, clients should be referred for evaluation for medication or inpatient treatment under the following conditions:

- When they are no longer benefiting from psychotherapy because they are too depressed to take consistent action to make cognitive, affective, and behavioral changes or so manic that their judgment is becoming unsound
- When they are too anxious to make progress using proven anxiety management techniques
- When their cognitions are loosely enough connected to confuse you, even after having established a therapeutic alliance
- When they are a high or rising suicide risk

Clients make slow or no progress in psychotherapy for a multitude of reasons. However, counselors, psychologists, and clients themselves often misinterpret why they seem stuck in therapy. Clients must be individually reassessed to determine whether they are merely resistant and malingering, whether the therapist is using the wrong techniques, or whether their lack of progress is being caused by underlying neuropsychological problems that drugs might well reduce. Our experience clearly indicates that many counselors and counseling psychologists see psychiatric medications as a last resort for failed therapy rather than as a complement to therapy that is in process. If psychotherapists do not learn the basics of pharmacopsychology and the actions of modern psychiatric drugs, this view will, unfortunately, be resistant to change.

A physician may ask the counselor for a recommendation on a drug to be prescribed, or a counselor may inadvertently offer such advice by referring the patient for an antidepressant rather than for an evaluation for depression. Counselors should decline to make such recommendations unless they are specifically trained as pharmacology consultants as they would be operating beyond the scope of their expertise and are legally liable for such advice. In many cases, physicians routinely make note of such advice in the patient's record, an act that may serve to establish a legal bridge to the counselor if the patient suffers harm from the drug.

By gaining knowledge in the field of pharmacopsychology, counselors learn that one drug can have many uses or indications. For example, a client who is prescribed an antidepressant medication (AM) may not be depressed but may have been prescribed an AM for chronic pain; Chapter 2 enumerates other uses for antidepressant drugs. Pharmaceutical companies not only introduce new drugs into the market but they also invest their resources testing new uses for established drugs. Counselors familiar with appropriate uses for particular medications are not as likely to mistakenly assume why a client is prescribed a particular drug.

Finally, it must be emphasized that psychiatric medications are not a magic bullet. They do not simply go to the center of the problem and destroy it. Medications reach throughout the body and affect most of its systems. Side effects are the product of this lack of specificity. Psychiatric medications do not exactly imitate the neurotransmitters whose actions they were designed to mimic and may produce other, though usually less severe, psychiatric symptoms. Further, individuals respond very differently to different drugs and different levels of drugs. Both drug and dose must fit the patient. During the early adjustment period, while side effects are most evident, medication management between physician and patient is most fragile. It is during this period of change that clients need the most support and counselors need the most expertise.

Likewise, it is during periods of disciplinary change that counselors have the most difficulty coping with new directions in their field. This book is designed to facilitate movement through this developmental period not only with clients but within the counseling discipline itself as pharmacopsychology takes its place as a necessary area of study.

1

THE NEUROLOGICAL BASIS
OF MENTAL DISORDERS

Faulty neurological function, often represented by defects in neurotransmitter activity, may result in emotional or mental disorders that are not fully comprehensible to counselors without an introductory knowledge of neuropharmacology and pharmacopsychology. Further, clients often want and need to understand the broad outlines of what their medications accomplish and why they experience neurological effects and side effects. If counselors do not have a clear understanding themselves, they cannot instruct their clients. Thus, demystification for both counselors and clients is the primary focus of this chapter. We hope this discussion will pique your interest in this area and serve as a basis to move ahead into reading or course work emphasizing what has become an explosion of information in neuropsychology and pharmacopsychology. Those who want a more detailed presentation of these topics should consult *A Primer of Drug Action* (Julien, 1992) and progress to *The Biochemical Basis of Neuropharmacology* (Cooper, Bloom, & Roth, 1991); both are well updated and accessible by independent study.

REGULATING EMOTION

Neurotransmission does not merely exercise strategic control over the processes of thinking, feeling, behaving, and the integration of the three; from our perspective it *is* these processes. They are inseparably bound. Each is the transitional end point of a complex neural process elaborated through 30 million years of primate evolution resulting in the ability of Homo sapiens to comprehend themselves and their world. Our design ensures that the brain is not static but can adapt (not always positively) its internal operations to utilize new and novel substances. Thus, the brain is less like a computer than it is like a vast, self-reflective chemistry set, parts of which are dedicated to routine maintenance operations and parts of which are dedicated to novel applications, depending on whether stimuli are from inside or outside the system. When the chemistry set under-, over-, or wrongly produces necessary constituents for neural activity, the system can be adjusted roughly through use of modern medicines that mimic or imitate properties of neurotransmitters. However, it must be emphasized that the adjustment is approximate and that side effects can restrict and negate even the positive aspects of the drug for many individuals. Given the dramatic increase in research on neuroactive drugs, it is clear that future psychiatric medications will allow neurotransmission to be much more finely tuned than we find possible today.

Neurotransmitters (NT), the primary chemical messengers in the brain, interact with one another and with neuromodulators and hormones to provide the two most important aspects of neural activity. The first is arousal, involving regulation of activity and rest. The second is orientation to time, place, and person, which are the fundamental aspects of consciousness. Arousal and orientation are controlled through the interplay of neurotransmitters that often work in opponent process to one another and in combination with regulatory neuropeptides (long chains of amino acids), sometimes called **neuromodulators (NM). Opponent process** implies that inhibitory and excitatory neurotransmitters, supported by peptide regulation, are in dynamic equilibrium within many systems of the brain. As excitatory activity rises, inhibitory or modulatory activity also rises so that excitation does not spiral out of control. An example of poorly regulated firing occurs in epilepsy where overfiring may be reflected in seizures. Further, there is a division of labor within the principal neurotransmitters such that

- some appear more devoted to excitatory processes (norepinephrine),
- some are more devoted to inhibition (gamma-aminobutyric acid),
- many (possibly most) are either excitatory or inhibitory depending on where they are found in the brain (dopamine), and
- some appear to be more regulatory in their effects on specific brain subsystems.

Dopamine and serotonin, for example, appear to up- or down-regulate the sensitivity of receptors to norepinephrine while at the same time performing more independent excitatory, inhibitory, or orientation functions within closely related neural systems (Cooper et al., 1991).

A general rule, the biological amine hypothesis of depression, to which there are, of course, many exceptions, is that depression can be equated roughly with a lack of excitatory neurotransmitters (or an inability to process them effectively) or an overabundance of neurotransmitters whose function is to inhibit neurotransmission. After a period of prolonged excitement or activity, many of us experience a bit of a low or depression that comes from exhaustion of excitatory neurotransmitters available in the neural net. Exhaustion of excitatory NTs, from chronic anxiety or worry or lengthy mental activity, can result in chronic depression that usually lifts once the work–rest system is in better equilibrium. However, individuals whose brains continue to produce insufficient levels of excitatory neurotransmitters or who are on medications that restrict that development or whose mental life has profoundly fatigued the system may become so chronically or profoundly depressed that they need medication. These latter forms of depression and accompanying depressed physical states are often treated with drugs that either mimic or raise the available levels of excitatory neurotransmitters within the brain.

Chronically high levels of excitement or mania and anxiety are treated with drugs that either tend to lower the level of excitatory neurotransmitters or raise the levels of or enhance the system's sensitivity to inhibitory neurotransmitters. The efficacy of this treatment strategy is further demonstrated by the fact that illegal or unwise use of drugs that inhibit the availability or activity of excitatory neurotransmitters (alcohol and other sedative hypnotics, for example) typically cause depression.

Similarly, although regulatory neurotransmitter functioning is intimately bound together with all the other neurotransmitters and neuromodulators, an excess of the (generally excitatory) NT dopamine or oversensitivity to dopamine is known to cause symptoms of psychosis, including disorganization of thought and behavior and, often, paranoia. Conversely, a deficiency of dopamine in the brain has been implicated in overly organized, stereotypic behaviors and autism.

Most of the NTs and NMs are found to activate and orient particular areas of the limbic system and the hypothalamus, areas of the brain whose duties include regulation of our emotional lives. Thus, a brief sketch of the nervous system and an in-depth look at neurotransmitters is the focus of the remainder of this first chapter.

THE NERVOUS SYSTEM

The nervous system consists of two major divisions. The central nervous system (CNS) includes the brain and spinal cord. The peripheral nervous system (PNS) includes all the nervous tissue outside the CNS. (For a brief outline of the structures of the CNS and the PNS, see the appendix.) The nervous system contains two basic cell types: neurons and glial cells.

NEURONS

Neurons are highly specialized nerve cells that conduct impulses throughout the brain and the body. Like all animal cells, neurons contain these features.

Cell membrane: the outer covering of a neuron composed of a double layer of **lipid** (fat-like) molecules. Many protein molecules float inside the lipid membrane. Protein molecules inside the membrane have special functions, such as detecting specific substances and relaying information about these substances and functioning as pumps to push out or pull in particles.

Nucleus: contains chromosomes (genetic material), which are long strands of DNA, and ribosomes, which function in protein synthesis. Proteins are important not only because they provide cell structure but also because they serve as **enzymes.** Enzymes act as catalysts for chemical reactions in both the synthesis and degradation of molecules. Specific enzymes catalyze specific processes.

Cytoplasm: a jelly-like substance that occupies space inside the neuron.

Many other particles are also found in a neuron. However, only the neural components important for understanding pharmacology are mentioned here.

Neurons exist in many shapes and varieties. The special purpose of a neuron determines its shape. Most neurons have four structures or regions:

Soma: the cell body of the neuron in which the nucleus and other vital components of the neuron reside.

Dendrite: the branching area of nerve cells. This dividing structure is similar to the branching of a tree. Dendrites and areas on the soma contain **receptors,** which are molecules that receive and react to messages from other neurons. The point where two neurons meet and relay information is called a **synapse.** Areas between neurons in which chemicals are transmitted are referred to as the **synaptic gap** or **synaptic cleft.**

Axon: a long slender tube of the neuron that relays electrical impulses from the soma to the terminal buttons of the neuron. The length of axons vary, ranging from a few millimeters in the brain to a meter in the spinal track. In the CNS, axons belonging to neurons of one region tend to group together and project to other areas of the brain. These CNS axon bundles are referred to as fibers or nerve fibers. Outside the CNS, the term *nerve* is used to describe bundles of axons.

Terminal buttons: Small knob-like structures at the end of axon clusters. Axons divide into numerous sub-axons, and each of these branches of axons end with a terminal button. **Vesicles** or small sacs inside terminal buttons contain chemicals (neurotransmitters) that are released after a relayed impulse reaches the end of the axon.

GLIAL CELLS

Glial cells, also referred to as neuroglia, are support cells of the nervous system. Glial cells serve various functions, including those listed here.

Hold the CNS together (like glue). Glial cells form a matrix to keep neurons in place.

Protect neurons. Glial cells physically and chemically buffer neurons. CNS neurons can be destroyed by head injury, infection, stroke, or other insults. When a neuron dies, it cannot be replaced, therefore the protective assistance of glial cells is important.

Clean up particles of dead cells.

Insulate neurons from other neurons. By surrounding and isolating synapses, glial cells aid in preventing neural messages from being scrambled.

Produce **myelin sheaths.** A myelin sheath is a series of segments forming a tube around the axon of a neuron. Myelin is composed of 80 percent lipid (fat) and 20 percent protein.

In the PNS, Schwann cells produce myelin to support and protect peripheral nerve cells. If a PNS axon is damaged, Schwann cells grow a protective tube to help direct new sprouts of the axon to muscles and sense organs. Unfortunately, glial cells in the CNS cannot perform the same task to repair damaged CNS neurons. CNS glial cells produce scar tissue that blocks reconnection of new sprouts.

BLOOD-BRAIN BARRIER

Years ago a psychologist found that a trypan dye injected into an animal's bloodstream would tint all blood tissues except the brain and spinal cord. Yet, if the dye were injected into the brain's ventricles, the blue dye would spread throughout the CNS.

The **blood-brain barrier (BBB)** is responsible for not allowing the dye to disperse from the blood into the brain tissues. This barrier between the circulating blood in the brain and the fluid that surrounds the brain tissue is composed of astrocytes, a type of glial cell that forms the physical basis of the BBB by encapsulating the capillaries in the brain.

The BBB is selectively permeable; that is, some substances (or drugs) gain entry to the CNS easily and others do not. Substances vital to the survival of neurons easily cross the BBB because of an active transport process. **Lipophilic molecules,** those that dissolve readily in fats (for example, those with low ionization), move effortlessly through the BBB. Alcohol is a lipophilic that not only can permeate the brain but also permeates the cells and nuclei of cells in the brain, where it acts as a toxin.

COMMUNICATION BETWEEN NEURONS

Neurons, of which there are approximately 20 billion in the brain, communicate with other neurons by way of chemicals called neurotransmitters. In the synaptic cleft, chemical neurotransmitters produce either an excitatory or inhibitory message on the receiving neuron. An excitatory message increases the likelihood that an impulse will be relayed, and an inhibitory message decreases the possibility that the impulse will be transmitted. All neurons can receive both excitatory and inhibitory impulses simultaneously. Therefore, whether a neuron relays a message down its axon depends on the relative activity (number) of the excitatory and inhibitory messages it receives.

One neuron can have tens of thousands of synapses on its membrane, allowing a neuron to be the recipient of information from many different neurons. This influx of information along as many as fifty thousand dendrites from various sources into one neuron is called **convergence.**

Generally, a neuron has only one axon; however, an axon branches into as many as ten thousand terminal buttons. Axonal branching is most profuse in the brain and most elaborate there in the memory systems. When an impulse is transmitted down the axon, it is conveyed to all axial branches. This branching allows a neuron to simultaneously send information to many other neurons, creating **divergence** of information.

ELECTRICAL PROPERTIES OF A NEURON.   A neuron's electrical charge is attributed to the difference in intracellular (within the neuron) and extracellular (outside the neuron) ion concentrations. **Ions** are small electrically charged molecules. Extracellular fluid is rich in sodium ions (symbolized as Na+) and chloride ions (C1-) and the intracellular fluid is rich in potassium (K+) and protein ions (A-). In a neuron's unexcited state, the average electrical difference between the intracellular and extracellular fluid is 70 millivolts (mV). The term *resting potential* is used to describe a neuron's unexcited state. The electrical charge when a neuron is at its resting potential is -70 mV.

ION EXCHANGE.   Recall that a neuron's membrane is a double layer of lipid molecules, called a *fluid mosaic,* that helps maintain the intracellular–extracellular ion concentration gradient. Molecules inside the neural membrane act as ion pumps or ion channels. When activated, these ion channels allow passage of specific ions (like neurotransmitters or drugs) across a membrane.

Two types of ion channels, differing in method of activation, exist in the neural membrane. The *voltage-dependent ion channel* is activated by changes in the membrane's electrical potential. The *neurotransmitter-dependent ion channel* is activated when neurotransmitters stimulate receptors that directly or indirectly open specific ion gates. Four types of neurotransmitter-dependent ion channels are known. Each causes either an inhibitory or excitatory response. They are:

- sodium (excitatory),
- chloride (inhibitory),
- potassium (excitatory), and
- calcium (excitatory) ion channels.

Activation of a specific ion channel is determined by both the particular neurotransmitter and the specific postsynaptic receptor that signals the ion channel to open (Carlson, 1991; Cooper et al., 1991).

CHANGE IN RESTING POTENTIAL.   A neurotransmitter causes a receiving neuron's electrical charge to become either *more negative*, a process called **hyperpo-**

larization, which produces an inhibitory effect by stabilizing the neural membrane, or *more positive*, a process called **depolarization**, which produces an excitatory effect. Hyperpolarizations are also called **inhibitory postsynaptic potentials (IPSPs)**. Depolarizations are also referred to as **excitatory postsynaptic potentials (EPSPs)**.

COMMUNICATION WITHIN A NEURON

The dendrite is the part of the neuron that branches off toward other cells and receives messages from them. At the dendrite, an activated neurotransmitter-dependent ion channel facilitates a change in intracellular ion concentration. Alterations in the intracellular ion concentration produce either the excitatory (EPSP) or the inhibitory effect (IPSP). The magnitude of the neuron's electrical change is proportional to the degree of stimulation on the neurotransmitter-dependent ion channel. Thus, the more NTs stimulate a postsynaptic dendrite, the greater the likelihood of producing an electrical change.

All EPSPs and IPSPs originating at the dendrites are averaged with all IPSPs or EPSPs generated from synapses directly on the soma or cell body. If a neuron's excitation synapses exert more influence than its inhibitory synapses, an **action potential (AP)** will be initiated at the axon hillock, the point where the neuron's axon connects to its soma. An AP is produced when a neuron's resting potential becomes less negative. The change in the resting potential has to reach a specific level or threshold before generating an AP.

All APs are the same size, yet not all behavioral responses are equal in magnitude. Stronger environmental stimuli produce a higher rate of firing of APs. For example, a bright light or loud sound may cause many APs to fire in a short time period, whereas a weak light or sound may stimulate fewer APs in the same time frame. The higher the firing rate of APs, the stronger the behavioral response will be (Carlson, 1991).

The AP is transmitted toward the axon's terminal buttons. Once it is at the axon's terminal button (or nerve end), the AP causes calcium ion channels in the neural membrane to open, allowing an influx of calcium ions ($Ca++$) to the neuron's terminal button. This influx of calcium ions causes vesicles or small reservoirs filled with neurotransmitter to merge with the membrane and release the neurotransmitters into the synaptic cleft. This process of releasing neuro-transmitters is called **exocytosis.**

In the synapse, neurotransmitters diffuse across the extracellular fluid and attach to postsynaptic receptors located on the adjacent neuron's soma or dendrite. At the postsynaptic dendrite or soma, neurotransmitters activate special molecules called receptors. Activating a receptor directly or indirectly opens ion channels in the postsynaptic neural membrane, which call for either excitation or inhibition. Recall that the passage of ions across a neural membrane will cause either hyperpolarization (inhibitory message) or depolarization (excitatory message).

RECEPTOR ACTIVATION.   All neurotransmitters fit into their respective receptors in a way similar to a key in a lock. There are two basic ways a neurotransmitter can open an ion channel. One way is through an acetylcholine receptor. When two acetylcholine (ACh) molecules occupy the two ACh sites on a single receptor, a sodium ion pump is opened, allowing an influx of sodium ions, which produces depolarization (and, therefore, excitation).

The second way an NT can open an ion channel is less direct and more complicated. A neurotransmitter (norepinephrine, for example) can attach to a receptor site, indirectly activating the production of cyclic adenosine monophosphate (cyclic AMP). Cyclic AMP, acting as a second messenger, activates enzymes (molecules that weaken or break down other substances) called protein kinases. In turn, protein kinases facilitate a change in the physical shape of proteins that control the opening of an ion channel. The alteration in the physical shape of the protein permits the opening, allowing an influx of ions into the postsynaptic neuron. This ion influx can cause either depolarization or hyperpolarization.

TERMINATION OF ACTIVITY IN THE SYNAPSE.   Postsynaptic potentials are brief. The neurotransmitter's work in the synaptic cleft occurs in a very short period of time, as quickly as one ten-thousandths of a second. Two mechanisms halt the action of neurotransmitters in the synapse; they are reuptake and enzymatic deactivation.

Reuptake is a process of extremely rapid removal of the neurotransmitter from the synaptic cleft by the presynaptic neuron's terminal button. **Enzymatic deactivation** is a degradation process of the neurotransmitter by an enzyme. For example, acetylcholine is destroyed by the enzyme acetylcholinesterase. And catecholamines are broken down for reuptake into the terminal vesicles by the enzymes monoamine oxidase (MAO) and catechol O-methyltransferase (COMT). (Note that enzymes usually end in the suffix -ase.)

CHARACTERISTICS OF NEUROTRANSMITTERS

Neurotransmitters and neuromodulators are chemicals that facilitate communication between neurons. NTs differ from NMs in that NMs are released from vesicles in greater quantities than NTs and can travel to other synapses in the brain. NTs usually act in the synapse where they are released.

Box 1-1   Life Cycle of an Endogenous Neurotransmitter

1. Neurotransmitters (NTs) are synthesized in the neuron.
2. Inside the neuron, NTs are stored in vesicles or small sacs in axon terminal buttons.
3. NTs are released from the neuron into the synapse by a process called exocytosis.
4. NTs exert their effect on the postsynaptic neuron.
5. NTs are released by the postsynaptic neuron back into the synapse.
6. NTs are deactivated either by enzymatic degradation or by the reuptake process **(endocytosis)** of the presynaptic neuron. [Julien, 1992]

In 1904, adrenalin (epinephrine) was the first NT to be described in the literature. Today, much information has been accumulated about NTs; however, many unknowns still exist. For example, researchers are not certain whether one neuron produces and releases several different NTs, although it is thought that each neuron produces a primary NT. Variants of that primary NT can, however, lock onto subsets of receptors, and a variety of neuroactive peptides (or NMs in some cases) can interact to condition the interaction of release and binding on the postsynaptic receptor. Scientists continue to identify new endogenous NTs and neuroactive peptides. Some NTs seem to be exclusively excitatory or inhibitory (the amino acid transmitter glycine, for example). Yet other NTs are capable of both inhibition and excitation (dopamine, for example) depending on the nature of the postsynaptic receptor an NT activates.

Neurotransmitters are commonly classified into four groups:

1. **Catecholamines,** so named because these NTs are derived from a compound called catechol and have an amine group. NTs included in this group are dopamine (DA), norepinephrine (NE), and epinephrine (Epi).
2. **Monoamines,** a more inclusive grouping system. The only criterion for membership in this class of NTs is belonging to a single amine group. All the catecholamines are also members of the monamine class, which consists of dopamine, norepinephrine, epinephrine, and serotonin or 5-hydroxytryptamine (5-HT).
3. **Amino acids,** building blocks for proteins. Amino acids also act as neurotransmitters in the CNS. Important amino acids include: gama-aminobutyric acid (GABA), glycine, and glutamic acid (glutamate).
4. **Neuropeptides,** chains of amino acids. Included in this group are endorphins and substance P.

MAJOR NEUROTRANSMITTERS

Acetylcholine (ACh) is neither a catecholamine nor a monoamine. ACh has major roles in both the PNS and the CNS. In the PNS, ACh is found at synapses where axons meet skeletal muscles. At this location, ACh causes excitation leading to muscle contraction. ACh is also widely distributed in the brain. Organic diseases in which ACh is thought to play an important role are Parkinson's disease, Alzheimer's disease, and myasthenia gravis.

Parkinson's disease, a movement disorder, is thought to result from an imbalance of DA and ACh in the basal ganglia of the brain. Dopaminergic neurons (cells that produce DA) degenerate in Parkinson's, resulting in ACh exerting a greater influence than DA. Sometimes, Parkinson's disease is treated with anticholinergic agents (drugs that decrease the action of ACh).

On the other hand, myasthenia gravis, a progressive disease of muscular weakness and fatigability, results from inadequate action of ACh. Myasthenia gravis is treated with drugs called cholinesterase inhibitors. Cholinesterase inhibitors suppress the action of the enzyme that breaks down ACh in synapses, thus prolonging the effects of ACh. Cholinesterase inhibitors are often used commercially as insecticides (which can have serious nervous system health consequences for humans who interact with them) and have been and are still employed on humans as lethal nerve gases.

Alzheimer's disease, a progressive disease that results in severe dementia and eventual death, has been associated with a deficiency in brain ACh. Memory deficits noted in Alzheimer's are thought to result, at least partially, from lower ACh levels in the hippocampus (Gossel & Wuest, 1992).

ACh is not only important for proper memory functioning but also plays a role in learning, behavioral arousal, attention, mood, and rapid eye movement (REM) activity that occurs during sleep. Drugs that mimic ACh or potentiate ACh effects facilitate REM sleep.

Epinephrine (Epi) is produced by the adrenal gland, a small endocrine gland located above the kidney. Epi exerts most of its effects in the PNS, where it functions to maintain heart rate and blood pressure. Epi is active in the brain but is not as important in neurotransmission as norepinephrine. **Adrenalin** is another term used for Epi.

Norepinephrine (NE) is primarily an excitatory NT. In the CNS, cell bodies of neurons that produce NE are located in the brain stem, with their axons projecting into the limbic system (a group of brain structures involved in emotions) and into the frontal lobes. NE is also involved in maintaining wakefulness and alertness. In the PNS, NE is active in "fight or flight" responses. When released in the spinal cord, NE exerts an analgesic effect by slowing the release of an NT called **substance P,** which activates pain reception.

Dopamine (DA) can produce both excitatory and inhibitory effects in the CNS. DA is thought to be involved in movement, learning, and attention. As described earlier, Parkinson's disease is caused by a deficiency of DA. One treatment for Parkinson's disease is to administer the drug L-dopa, a precursor to DA. L-dopa can cross the BBB, while DA can not. Once in the brain, some of the L-dopa is converted to DA. Overactivity of DA or oversensitivity of DA receptors is linked with symptoms of schizophrenia. Parkinson's patients treated with L-dopa occasionally have side effects similar to symptoms of schizophrenia. And, in the same vein, side effects of phenothiazine drugs (which deplete DA and are, therefore, used in treatment of schizophrenia), often produce the involuntary movements characteristic of Parkinson's disease.

Two types of DA receptors have been isolated, called D1 and D2. Amphetamine and cocaine, two frequently abused drugs, activate DA receptors; this activation of DA receptors produces stimulating and reinforcing properties (excitation) and also helps account for the schizophrenia-like behaviors common to large-scale or long-term use of these drugs.

Serotonin (5-HT) is thought to be involved in the inhibition of activity and behavior. It is active in mood regulation, control of eating, sleep and arousal, and pain regulation. Axons of NE and 5-HT project into almost the same areas of the brain; NE and 5-HT are thought to have opposing actions in these areas. Antidepressant drugs, particularly the heterocyclics like fluoxetine (Prozac) and sertraline (Zoloft), work principally by blocking the reuptake of 5-HT (Beasley, Masica, & Potvin, 1992; Reimherr et al., 1990; Stahl, 1992).

Gamma-aminobutyric acid (GABA) is an amino acid that functions as an inhibitory NT by making the brain more stable and preventing overexcitation of neurons. Several sedating drugs, such as the benzodiazepines and barbiturates, are active at GABA receptor site complexes.

Glutamate is an excitatory amino acid NT that lowers the threshold for neural excitation. It is often in oriental food in the form of monosodium glutamate. After ingesting large quantities of glutamate, individuals sensitive to glutamate may experience dizziness and other transient but mild neurological symptoms.

Glycine is another amino acid. Glycine has inhibitory effects in the spinal cord, where it is highly concentrated. The poison strychnine blocks glycine, thus preventing glycine's inhibitory action, resulting in continual seizures. If an antidote for this poison is not administered quickly, death usually results (Klaassen, 1993).

Neuropeptides, or neuromodulators, unlike amino acid and monoamine NTs that come from dietary sources, are produced within cells in ribosomes where their synthesis is directed by messenger RNA (mRNA). Neuropeptides are composed of chains of amino acids and are intermediate between amino acids and proteins in size.

Endorphins or **opioid peptides** are internally manufactured neuropeptides that, like morphine after which they are named, can produce analgesia, affect the perception of pain, induce respiratory depression, cause sedation, and alter affective behavior and feelings of well-being. **Enkephalins** and **dynorphins** are other terms used to refer to subgroups of these neuromodulators.

As there are different varieties of endorphins, various types of CNS endorphin receptors exist. Opioid NMs are very specific molecules, meaning that only specific NMs can stimulate certain opioid receptors. The chemical structure of the opioid NM will determine which receptor it can activate.

PHARMACOLOGY IN THE NEURON

Drugs can alter behavior by interrupting or altering any one of the many processes that occur in neural communication. A drug that increases the availability or mimics the action of an endogenous NT is called an **agonist**. Conversely, a drug that decreases the availability or action of an NT is called an **antagonist**. Agonist drug actions include

- being a precursor for an NT, resulting in an increase in NT synthesis,
- increasing release of NTs from terminal buttons,
- acting like endogenous NTs and stimulating postsynaptic receptors,
- blocking reuptake by presynaptic neurons, allowing NTs to remain in synapse longer, and
- immobilizing enzymes that break down NTs in synapse, thus increasing the number of NTs in the synapse available for action. [Carlson, 1991]

Antagonist drug actions include

- decreasing the production of an NT by blocking the enzyme required for its synthesis,
- blocking storage of NTs in vesicles,
- preventing release of NTs from terminal buttons,
- binding postsynaptic receptors without stimulating them, hindering NT activity, and
- stimulating receptors on presynaptic neurons, called autoreceptors, which tell neurons not to release NTs. [Carlson, 1991]

CONCLUSION

We hope this outline of the fundamentals of neurotransmission will enhance your understanding of the discussions presented in the chapters that follow. In reading those chapters, bear in mind that as we achieve a deeper understanding of neurophysiology, we increase our knowledge of the psychiatric problems that accompany faulty neurotransmission.

2

DEPRESSION AND ANTIDEPRESSANTS

BIPOLAR DISORDER AND LITHIUM

This chapter provides an introduction to the underlying somatic and emotional causes of depression and discusses the relationship between its etiology and its treatment. We will pay special attention to the issues of why, when, and how counselors should refer clients to a physician for evaluation concerning antidepressant medication. Finally, we will discuss what is known of the etiology of bipolar disorder (also called manic-depression), the psychiatric drugs used in its treatment, and the drug compliance problems that often arise.

DEPRESSION

Depression is the second most common psychiatric disorder in adults, following anxieties. Depression, however, is a more life-threatening emotional illness and accounts for approximately 75 percent of psychiatric hospitalizations; 20 percent of women and 10 percent of men experience at least one major depressive episode in their lives (Fuller & Underwood, 1989). The potential danger of depression is illustrated by the fact that severely depressed patients are at high risk for suicide. Approximately 80 percent of suicidal individuals have depressive illnesses.

Depression is considered to be a mood illness, whereas schizophrenia, for example, is a disease primarily interfering with perception and thought processes. However, schizophrenia often does produce severe secondary depressive episodes. These secondary depressive episodes may produce active psychoses in 10 to 15 percent of depressed clients with schizophrenia (Jonas & Schaumburg, 1991).

DIAGNOSIS

The *Diagnostic and Statistical Manual of Mental Disorders, Fourth Edition* (DSM-IV) (American Psychiatric Association, 1994) describes the criteria for a diagnosis of depression. Feelings of depressed mood or loss of pleasure in almost all activities that lasts for at least two weeks is the essential feature of a major unipolar depressive episode.

Depressed clients are often unable to cope and are immobilized without understanding why. They often feel guilty for their lack of self-efficacy and self-esteem and are shamed by their condition. This sense of shame further restricts their range of social interactions, which further reinforces their view of themselves as inadequate.

Although the average age of onset for depression is late 20s, it may occur much earlier (APA, 1994). Depression in children, as in the elderly, is less well researched (Waterman & Ryan, 1993), often misdiagnosed, and underreported. The link between many childhood behavioral disorders (attention-deficit hyper-activity disorder, for example) and depression is only now being explored (Gadow, 1992; Klein, 1987). For an update on attention-deficit hyperactivity disorders (ADHD), see Pelham (1993). Further, exploration of the relationship between chronic pain, chronic fatigue, and depression among adults has also been neglected until very recently. These conditions are clearly interconnected.

UNIPOLAR DEPRESSION SUBTYPES

Unipolar depression encompasses a large group of heterogenous conditions that include major depression, dysthymia, and minor depression. A broad distinction can be made among the many depression classification systems. The depression subtypes *biological, endogenous,* and *primary* can be contrasted with another cluster of depression types that include *reactive, situational, exogenous,* and *secondary* (Lawson & Copperrider, 1988). As implied by the names, the etiology or precipitating factors are somewhat different between the two broad groupings. The former cluster is suspected to occur because of a spontaneous biochemical imbalance in the brain and is thought to have a genetic basis, even though environmental triggers, such as stress, may exist. This genetic predisposition plus its triggering mechanism is often referred to as a *stress-diathesis model* of depression. The latter cluster of depression types is considered to be a secondary response to external events such as personal loss, financial problems, health problems, or administration of certain medications. Swonger and Matejski (1991) estimate that 20 percent of the cases of major depressive episodes are endogenous and 80 percent are exogenous. Interestingly, the symptoms and recovery rates for situational and nonsituational depressions are comparable, even though the relapse rate and lethality appears higher in endogenous depression (Hammen, 1991).

DYSTHYMIA. A further important subdivision of unipolar depression is the distinction drawn in DSM-IV between major depression, which is either episodic and acute (or even seasonal), and *dysthymia* or depressive neurosis. **Dysthymia** is a subacute form of depression that is continuous for a minimum of two years (one year in children). Its symptoms are present without breaks of more than two months, and it is chronic. Dysthymia, like major depression, is thought to be both endogenously and exogenously caused. Symptoms of major depression are either not present in dysthymia, not present for long, or are in remission. The client often feels fatigue, low self-esteem, hopelessness, and may have either a poor appetite or overeat. The client may have insomnia or hypersomnia, poor concentration, or have difficulty making decisions. Dysthymia is often divided into two groups: primary and secondary. Primary dysthymia is not caused by other DSM-IV Axis I nonmood disorders (for example, schizophrenia or substance abuse) or by Axis III medical disorders. Secondary dysthymia is thought to be caused by a chronic DSM-IV Axis I or Axis III disorder.

Dysthymic individuals found to have a major depressive episode are said to suffer from **double depression** and are high risks for suicide.

MINOR DEPRESSION. Minor depression includes dysthymia, cyclothymia, depression not otherwise specified, and adjustment disorder with depressed mood. These conditions are good candidates for antidepressant drug treatment *if psychotherapy has not made a significant difference in the level of depression after three months* (Stewart, Quitkin, & Klein, 1992).

DRUGS THAT PRODUCE DEPRESSION. Some drugs are known to produce exogenous or secondary types of depression (see Box 2-1). Therapists should pay special attention to all drugs their clients are taking, including over-the-counter (OTC) and abusable drugs that may cause depression or other psychiatric conditions.

It is also common for depression to occur secondarily to biological disease processes. Numerous illnesses can precipitate a depressive state. A list of the more common medical conditions associated with depression is included in Box 2-2.

ETIOLOGY

The **biological amine hypothesis of depression** states that there is a functional deficit of the neurotransmitters serotonin (5-HT) or norepinephrine (NE) in the brain. This hypothesis is supported by the fact that antidepressants increase levels of NE and 5-HT along with alleviating many of the signs and symptoms of depression. Other evidence offered as support for this hypothesis is that drugs like reserpine, which lower blood pressure, also lower central nervous system levels of NE and 5-HT and produce depression. Further support is provided from

Box 2-1   Drugs Associated with Exogenous Depression

Sedative–Hypnotic Agents
Alcohol
Benzodiazepines (see Chapter 3)
Barbiturates (see Chapter 3)
Equanil (meprobamate)
Noctec (chloral hydrate)

**Anti-Inflammatory and
Analgesic Agents**
Butazolidin (phenylbutazone)
Indocin (indomethacin)
Opioids or narcotics (see Chapter 5)
Talwin (pentazocine)

Steroids
Corticosteroids
Estrogen withdrawal
Oral contraceptives

Over-the-Counter Drugs
Antihistamines

Miscellaneous Agents
Antineoplastic agents (used for cancers)
Anti-Parkinson drugs (see Chapter 4)
Antipsychotic drugs (see Chapter 4)
Myambutal Ethambutol (used for tuberculosis)

Other Abusable Drugs
Marijuana
Opium derivatives (morphine, codeine)
Phencyclidine (PCP) (anesthetic psychedelic)

**Antihypertensive and
Cardiovascular Drugs**

Trade Name	Generic Name
Aldomet	Methyldopa
Apresoline	Hydralazine
Catapres	Clonidine
Inderal	Propranolol
Ismelin	Guanethidine
Lanoxin	Digoxin
Lopressor	Metoprolol
Minipress	Prazosin
Pronestyl	Procainamide
Serpasil	Reserpine

Sources: Fuller & Underwood, 1989; Olin et al., 1993; Taylor, 1990.

research that has shown mania (the behavioral opposite of depression) to result from an overabundance of NE in the synaptic cleft.

However, it is suspected that the biological amine model of depression is too simplistic. The reason for this suspicion is that although the effects of antidepressant medications (AMs) on brain levels of NE and 5-HT are immediate the reversal of depressive symptoms is delayed two to six weeks after the initiation of antidepressant therapy. A more sophisticated theory would explain the triggering and feedback systems in the brain that may account for the delayed action. It is reasonable to assume that the brain does not simply interpret a rise in arousal produced by excitatory neurotransmitters as an end to depression. Depression is a complex affective syndrome that includes low arousal, changes in the levels of a number of neurotransmitters responsible for both orientation and arousal, and individual interpretation of internal and external states. Further, our experience

---

Box 2-2 Medical Conditions Associated with Exogenous Depression

Endocrine Disorders
Addison's disease
Cushing's disease
Diabetes mellitus
Hyperparathyroidism
Hyperthyroidism
Hypothyroidism

Central Nervous System Disorders
Alzheimer's disease
Brain tumors
Huntington's disease
Multiple sclerosis
Parkinson's disease

Cardiovascular Disorders
Cerebral vascular accident (stroke)
Congestive heart failure
Myocardial infarction

Miscellaneous Disorders
Carcinoma (cancer)
Infectious disease
Malnutrition
Mental retardation
Metabolic abnormalities
Pancreatic disease
Pernicious anemia
Rheumatoid arthritis
Systemic lupus erythematosus

Sources: Fuller & Underwood, 1989; Taylor, 1990.

---

as therapists indicates that depressed individuals do not necessarily recognize the early movement out of depression, even though we may see clear changes in the client's mood, thinking, and behavior. It is therefore of great importance that we help clients accurately track their therapeutic movement and instill hope.

It is crucial to recognize that many suicides occur during phases when the client feels more capable of action (vegetative, physical symptoms are improving) but feels no less emotionally overwhelmed by the depression (nonvegetative symptoms are not improving). Attention should be focused for a definite period of time each session on suicide issues and, if necessary, on (control) contracts that include realistic crisis management steps.

Finally, and particularly warranted by continued deterioration of impulse control or substance abuse, orderly steps for inpatient treatment need to be discussed with the client.

TREATMENT OF DEPRESSION

Even though depression is the most common mental or emotional problem leading to psychotherapy, most people do not seek treatment (Hammen, 1991). Further, 60 percent of depressed persons who do seek treatment are misdiagnosed as suffering from other problems (Restak, 1988). Finally, among those who take antidepressant medications (AMs), 30 to 50 percent discontinue the drug before treatment effects can take place or are prescribed a dose below the effective treatment dosage (Kimberly et al., 1992).

Depression can impede physical, psychological, and social functioning. The combination of adverse physiological effects and emotional instability frequently lead depressed patients to suicidal ideation. Further, approximately 50 percent of people with a history of depression among first-degree relatives will have depressive episodes (Restak, 1988).

Studies comparing the efficacy of drug treatment for depression with psychotherapy have not found significant differences. However, bimodal treatment, which includes both psychotherapy and antidepressant medication (AM), improves the recovery rate for depression over and above either intervention used alone. Emotional coping and social functioning are aided primarily by psychotherapy, while the physiological symptoms are helped by antidepressants. The beneficial effects of exercise and diet on the physiological symptoms of depression should not be underestimated. For cases of severe depression that are unresponsive to drug treatment and psychotherapy, electroconvulsive therapy (ECT) is available.

Unmedicated episodes of major depression usually last between four and six months (APA, 1994). If a patient has two or more depressive episodes within a relatively short time period and has a history or family history of positive responses to antidepressant agents, then long-term prophylactic AM treatment may be warranted. **Prophylactic treatment** (treatment that generally lasts longer than one year and is given to forestall a relapse) should not be unsupervised for a variety of reasons. Side effects may, over time, begin to outweigh therapeutic effects of the drug. AMs are expensive, often costing more than $100 per month, and clients often weigh their therapeutic advantages against their costs. Newer, less toxic forms of AMs may soon be available.

REFERRAL CONSIDERATIONS.   Studies have shown that depression relapses occur when antidepressants are discontinued soon after the acute symptoms have been controlled (Hammen, 1991). Relapse is less likely to occur when AMs are discontinued several months after the acute symptoms have abated and after psychotherapy has begun. In their classic study, *The Cognitive Therapy of Depression*, Beck, Rush, Shaw, and Emery (1979) provide a list of characteristics to consider when deciding whether cognitive therapy, antidepressant therapy, or a combination of therapies should be undertaken (see Box 2-3). Although their discussion is directed at cognitive therapy options, other forms of psychotherapy shown to be effective in cases of depression may be generalized.

TREATMENT CONSIDERATIONS.   Counselors are routinely faced with several converging problems concerning clients and their use of depression medication. First, counselors are expected to understand the client's point of view regarding problems with their antidepressant. Second, counselors are expected to know the conditions under which clients should be referred to a physician for appraisal for AM. Third, counselors are expected to help clients with drug compliance. Fourth, counselors are expected to understand and educate the client about the interactions of their medication and alcohol or illicit drugs and issues of dual diagnosis.

MISCONCEPTIONS ABOUT DEPRESSION AND TREATMENT.   To increase compliance and educate the client, counselors need to explore misconceptions about the client's

Box 2-3   Choosing an Appropriate Plan for Therapy

Criteria that would justify administration of cognitive therapy alone

1. Failure to respond to adequate trials of two different AMs
2. Partial response to adequate doses of AMs
3. Failure to respond or only partial response to other psychotherapies
4. Diagnosis of minor affective disorder
5. Variable mood reactive to environmental events
6. Variable mood that correlates with negative cognitions
7. Mild somatic disturbance symptoms (sleep, appetite, weight, or libidinal)
8. Adequate reality testing (that is, no hallucinations or delusions) and adequate span of concentration and memory function
9. Inability to tolerate medication side effects, or evidence that excessive risk is associated with pharmacotherapy

Situations in which cognitive therapy alone is not indicated

1. Evidence of coexisting schizophrenia, organic brain syndrome, alcoholism, narcotic abuse, or mental retardation
2. Patient has medical illness or is taking medication likely to cause depression
3. Obvious memory impairment or poor reality testing (hallucinations, delusions)
4. History of manic episodes (bipolar depression)
5. History of family member who responded to antidepressant medication
6. History of family member with bipolar illness
7. Absence of precipitating or exacerbating environmental stresses
8. Little evidence of cognitive distortions
9. Presence of severe somatic complaints (for example, pain)

Situations in which medication plus cognitive therapy are appropriate

1. Partial or no response to a trial of cognitive therapy alone
2. Partial but incomplete response to adequate pharmacotherapy alone
3. Poor compliance with medication regimen
4. Historical evidence of chronic maladaptive functioning with depressive syndrome on an intermittent basis
5. Presence of severe somatic symptoms and marked cognitive distortions (for example, hopelessness)
6. Impaired memory and concentration and marked psychomotor difficulty
7. Severe depression with suicidal danger
8. History of first-degree relative who responded to antidepressants
9. History of mania in close relative or patient

Source: From *Cognitive Therapy of Depression* by A. Beck, A. J. Rush, B. F. Shaw, G. Emery, pp. 366–368, The Guilford Press, 1979. Reprinted by permission of Aaron Beck.

medications, depression, and psychotherapy. Beck et al. (1979) outlined the cognitions contributing to poor adherence to medication prescription (see Box 2-4).

Other misconceptions about AMs are that once AMs are begun they cannot be discontinued due to medical reasons, that the side effects are permanent, that the therapist is responsible for the depression management, that psychotherapy

---

Box 2-4   Client Cognitions Contributing to Poor Drug Compliance

Client cognitions about the medication before taking it

1. It's addicting.
2. I am stronger if I don't need medicine.
3. I am weak to need it (a crutch).
4. It won't work for me.
5. If I don't take medication, I'm not crazy.
6. I can't stand side effects.
7. I'll never get off medication once I start.
8. There's nothing I need to do except take medicine.
9. I only need to take medication on "bad days."

Client cognitions about the medication while taking it

1. Since I'm perfectly well (or not any better) after days or weeks, the medicine isn't working.
2. I should feel good right away.
3. The medicine will solve all my problems.
4. The medicine won't solve problems, so how can it help?
5. I can't stand the dizziness (or fuzziness) or other side effects.
6. It makes me into a zombie.

Client cognitions about depression

1. I am not ill (I don't need help).
2. Only weak people get depressed.
3. I deserve to be depressed since I am a burden on everybody.
4. Isn't depression a normal reaction to the bad state of things?
5. Depression is incurable.
6. I am one of the small percentage that does not respond to any treatment.
7. Life isn't worth living, so why should I try to get over my depression?

Source: From *Cognitive Therapy of Depression* by A. Beck, A. J. Rush, B. F. Shaw, G. Emery, p. 372, The Guilford Press, 1979. Reprinted by permission of Aaron Beck.

---

makes it possible to cut back (lower the dose) on the amount of AM, that therapy can completely and permanently cure depression, and that depression will change without clients examining and possibly changing how they think, act, and feel in a wide range of areas.

Because beliefs that sabotage successful therapy are often subtle and deeply held, coming from the family and from society at large, therapists must engage clients in a dialogue about their beliefs concerning their problems and possible solutions. A willingness and ability to confront these issues, of course, lies at the heart of why counselors are successful in treating depression. During active depression, clients' cognitions are often distorted so that education and rational appraisal of the situation is compromised. Clients are likely to selectively attend to accounts of the usefulness or harmfulness of the drugs they are using. They may unreasonably magnify the meaning and importance of side effects, and because their feedback systems are dulled, clients may be unaware of positive changes in their cognitions and overt behaviors. Counselors must, therefore, ask for client reports on their physical, emotional, and cognitive condition during each counseling session and direct the client toward an understanding of the meaning of these conditions to their overall progress. Counselors must work to keep the client aware of the progress being made without rescuing the client.

TREATMENT RESPONSE. A poorer response to medication is predicted for individuals who have experienced an abrupt onset to depression and have a history of depressive episodes that are of long duration. Biological and situational depressions appear to respond similarly to medication, especially the vegetative, somatic symptoms. Although psychotherapy is thought to affect most cognitive and emotional symptoms, the effects of AMs on mood and emotional symptoms should not be underestimated. Emotional pain is caused by changes in neurotransmission, particularly in the hypothalamus, not simply by painful thoughts.

Two of the most commonly prescribed groups of AMs (tricyclics and heterocyclics) have well-known side effects. Two tricyclics, amitriptyline (Elavil) and imipramine (Tofranil), raise blood pressure specifically. If the client has hypertension, either doxepin (Sinequan), a tricyclic antidepressant with low hypertensive qualities, or a heterocyclic second-generation AM may be prescribed. Counselors should be reminded that idiosyncratic (out-of-the-ordinary), paradoxical (reversed), toxic, and allergic reactions can occur with all drugs. Ask the client to arrange to have a medication evaluation if acute physical or divergent psychiatric problems persist.

REFERRAL. Depressed clients should be referred to a psychiatrist or family practice physician for appraisal for medications (or for possible hospitalization) when any one of these circumstances is present:

1. Client is at a high risk for suicide. Risk factors include patient history and family history of suicide or high-risk behaviors, present crisis, present depression inventories (Beck Depression Inventory, for example), risk demographics (age, sex, and isolation, for example), threatens to harm oneself, and has a feasible plan to implement suicidal actions.

2. Client exhibits intense vegetative signs, including early morning wakening, melancholia, somatic symptoms (weight loss, insomnia, agitation, or psychomotor restlessness, for example).

3. Client is psychotic (for example, client exhibits severe impairment in reality testing as manifested by hallucinations or delusions).

4. Client has a history of alcohol or other drug abuse or dependence.

5. Client has impairments to memory, attention, or signs of muscle weakness or spasticity.

6. There is evidence, as presented above, that there are sufficient reasons to include pharmacotherapy in the treatment regime, or if it is suspected that the client's present prescription drugs may be causing unwanted side effects.

It is important to note that AMs can cause the activation of *latent psychosis.* This appears especially true of the tricyclic AMs, which may raise the level of catecholamines, including dopamine, which are excitatory neurotransmitters. It is well known that schizophrenia is exacerbated by rises in the levels of dopamine and norepinephrine, and this problem may extend to other forms of psychosis as well. This activation of latent psychosis is considered less likely for the nontricyclic AMs, particularly those that differentially raise serotonin levels (for example, sertraline and fluoxetine).

COMPLIANCE.   Today, the number of depressed clients on AMs who arrive for psychotherapy is rising. Numerous reasons exist for this increase in AM usage. Physicians who prescribe AMs are becoming better educated to the drug compliance and long-term recovery benefits to their patients of combining AMs and psychotherapy, and therefore refer clients for counseling more readily. Given the reduced side effects (and lowered suicide risk) of second-generation heterocyclic AMs (a fluoxetine such as Prozac, for example), AMs are more likely to be prescribed for reactive depressive episodes. And physicians have a wider range of AMs to chose from when prescribing.

Counselors and other mental health workers need to be aware of clients' thinking processes that may affect their drug compliance. Clients not thoroughly educated on the issues of medication therapy may believe that since they are in psychotherapy they are no longer expected to continue their AMs. Further, depressed clients' thinking and listening processes concerning their medications may be distorted by their depression; thus, clients may not process clearly what is said to them. Finally, clients may be entering psychotherapy as an alternative to drug therapy without having discussed discontinuing their medications with their prescribing physicians.

CLASSES OF ANTIDEPRESSANTS
TRICYCLIC ANTIDEPRESSANTS

All **tricyclic antidepressants (TCAs)** have the same basic three-ring chemical structure and are related to the phenothiazine class of antipsychotics (Olin et al., 1993). TCAs are 65 to 75 percent effective in relieving the somatic features associated with depression, and TCAs have been shown to be effective in treating both exogenous and endogenous depression (Joyce & Paykel, 1989). TCAs are often prescribed for patients with decreased appetite, weight loss, early morning awakening, lack of interest in the people and objects in their environment, and a family history of depression combined with a history of responsiveness to medication. However, highly anxious, fearful, or phobic patients, who have many physical complaints and who haven't improved with an adequate trial of TCAs, may respond to monoamine oxidase inhibitors or second-generation heterocyclic AMs. It should be remembered that response to TCAs may differ by sex, although data on sexual differences in response to TCAs is conflicting. Even though a majority of TCAs are taken by women, most clinical trials have utilized male subjects (Dawkins & Potter, 1991).

MECHANISMS AND ACTIONS. TCA drugs exert their effects by blocking the reuptake of the excitatory neurotransmitters NE and, secondarily, 5-HT to the presynaptic membrane. Blocking the reuptake of these neurotransmitters causes an increase of NE and 5-HT in the synaptic cleft. One TCA, clomipramine (Anafranil) specifically prevents the reuptake of 5-HT, not NE (Trimble, 1990). Specific effects of TCAs include:

- mood elevation,
- increase in physical activity and mental alertness,
- improvement in sleep and appetite, and
- nonelevation of mood in nondepressed subjects. [American Medical Association, 1983]

PHARMACOKINETICS. TCAs are easily absorbed and are not affected by the intake of food. Because most TCAs have long elimination half-lives (time period it takes to excrete one half of the drug), TCAs can be administered just once a day (usually at bedtime). Metabolism occurs in the liver, and TCAs are excreted in the feces and urine. TCAs are highly protein bound. Being very lipid (fat) soluble, TCAs are easily distributed throughout the brain (Olin et al., 1993).

DRUG INTERACTIONS. Because they bind to plasma proteins in the blood stream, TCAs are at risk for numerous drug interactions. Drug interactions with TCAs can be severe, especially in the geriatric population, who often consume a wide range of medications. Drug interactions occur most frequently with drugs having sedative (benzodiazepine), anticholinergic (antihistamine), or hypotensive (blood pressure lowering) properties (Baldessarini, 1993).

SIDE EFFECTS. Side effects are common with TCA therapy. However, a tolerance for anticholinergic medications usually develops over time. The most common side effects are the following:

- Anticholinergic effects—especially common for people taking amitriptyline (Elavil) or imipramine (Tofranil): dry mouth (50 to 74 percent), blurred vision (6 to 20 percent), urinary retention, and constipation
- Cardiac arrhythmias
- Hypertension—especially common for people taking Elavil or Tofranil
- Sedation
- Hypotension or dizziness (18 to 52 percent)
- Other reversible side effects, such as seizures, insomnia, headache, tachycardia, tremor, and fatigue [Fuller & Underwood, 1989]

INTERACTIONS AND TOXICITY. TCAs have a narrow therapeutic window. An acute overdose with TCAs can be fatal. With high doses, TCAs can produce serious hypotension (drop in blood pressure) that can lead to cardiac arrhythmia and death. Because these arrhythmias are very difficult to treat, and because of their risk for use in suicide, it is recommended that an acutely depressed patient or a high-risk patient receive no more than a one-week supply of TCAs (Baldessarini, 1993).

DRUG SELECTION AND DOSING. Selection of a specific TCA is based upon a patient's drug response history, target symptoms, and the TCA's side effects. Table 2-1 outlines the common uses of various TCAs. Dosages of TCAs are individualized. The initial dosage for a TCA is usually one-third to one-half of the therapeutic dose. If the desired response is not obtained, the dose is increased gradually. Gradual dose increases help minimize adverse effects (Swonger & Matejski, 1991). Response to the drug occurs within 14 to 21 days, with the maximum effect appearing in four to six weeks. TCA therapy is not considered ineffective until a four-week trial is completed with no measurable effects (Olin et al., 1993).

TCAs are not reinforcing drugs; they do not produce euphoria or stimulate the brain's pleasure centers. Because of the delay in the desired effects and the

Table 2-1 Tricyclic Antidepressants and Their Uses

Trade Name	Generic Name	Other Uses
Adapin	Doxepin	Anxiety Chronic pain*
Anafranil	Clomipramine	Only obsessive-compulsive disorders (OCD) Chronic pain* Panic disorder*
Asendin	Amoxapine	
Aventyl	Nortriptyline	Panic disorder*
Elavil	Amitriptyline	Eating disorder* Chronic pain*
Endep	Amitriptyline	Eating disorder* Chronic pain*
Norpramin	Desipramine	Eating disorder* (bulimia) Facilitation of cocaine withdrawal*
Pamelor	Nortriptyline	Panic disorder*
Pertofrane	Desipramine	Eating disorder* (bulimia)
Sinequan	Doxepin	Anxiety Chronic pain*
Surmontil	Trimipramine	
Tofranil	Imipramine	Child enuresis Panic disorder* Eating disorder* (bulimia)
Vivactil	Protriptyline	

*Unlabeled use

Source: Olin et al., 1993.

immediate appearance of side effects with TCAs, patients may become discouraged and discontinue treatment. It is imperative (a) that patients be encouraged to continue treatment until the medication has had a chance to work, and (b) that patients be reassured that bothersome (anticholinergic) side effects of TCAs do not impose any serious problems and usually abate within several weeks. Anticholinergic side effects can also be controlled with Urecholine (bethanechol).

DISCONTINUATION. Although TCAs are not addictive, abrupt discontinuation following a prolonged period of treatment can produce unwanted symptoms, including nausea, headache, vertigo, nightmares, and malaise. A gradual withdrawal from treatment over two weeks will lessen these symptoms (Olin et al., 1993).

MONOAMINE OXIDASE INHIBITOR ANTIDEPRESSANTS

Monoamine oxidase inhibitor antidepressants (MAOIs) are indicated as treatment for depression in some patients who are unresponsive to other antidepressants. Due to their severe side effects and the potential for serious interaction with other drugs and foods, MAOIs are rarely used first as the drug of choice when treating depression. The relationship between MAOIs and food intake stems from the regulation of tyramine metabolism by MAO. When MAO is inhibited, the presence of tyramine in the system can precipitate a hypertensive crisis (Julien, 1992). MAOIs exert their effect by inhibiting the enzyme monoamine oxidase, which is responsible for the breakdown of neurotransmitters NE, 5-HT, and epinephrine, thereby increasing the levels of these neurotransmitters. The most common MAOIs are listed in Table 2-2. As with TCAs, there is usually a delay of several weeks in therapeutic action (Maxmen, 1991).

SIDE EFFECTS. Common side effects are postural hypotension (fall in blood pressure on standing), dizziness, headache, insomnia, fatigue, and tremors. Serious effects of MAOIs are liver damage and hypertensive crisis resulting from synergism with certain drugs and foods (Olin et al., 1993). This hypertension can be fatal, causing hemorrhaging in the brain.

DRUG INTERACTIONS AND TOXICITY. Many over-the-counter (OTC) products, such as cold and sinus medicine, present a serious hazard to patients taking MAOIs. The following are other drugs and foods that pose a serious threat if administered with or within two weeks of MAOI therapy.

Table 2-2 MAOI Antidepressants and Their Uses

Trade Name	Generic Name	Other Uses
Marplan	Isocarboxazid	
Nardil	Phenelzine	Treatment-resistant
Parnate	Tranylcypromine	Reactive depression

Source: Olin et al., 1993.

Drugs to Avoid When Taking MAOIs	Foods to Avoid When Taking MAOIs	
TCAs and heterocyclics	cheese	wine
Demerol (meperidine)	yogurt	beer
amphetamine stimulants	chocolate	cream
sympathomimetics	caffeine	pickled herring
tryptophan	fava beans	chicken liver

Because of possible toxic interactions with other antidepressants, MAOIs should be allowed sufficient time to clear the system before other AMs are begun. In some cases, this clearing period lasts four weeks in both directions (that is, MAOI cleared for non-MAOI, and non-MAOI cleared for use of MAOI).

HETEROCYCLIC ANTIDEPRESSANTS

The **second generation,** atypical or **heterocyclic antidepressants** are usually contrasted with the tricyclics or first generation AMs. Table 2-3 lists common heterocyclic antidepressants and their uses. Second generation antidepressants are somewhat less toxic and appear to have a more rapid onset than do tricyclics. They also appear to produce fewer side effects, especially anticholinergic effects. As a general rule, heterocyclic antidepressants produce less weight gain, less sedation and hypotension, and appear potentially useful in treating obsessive-compulsive repetitive or stereotypy symptoms and eating disorders (McBride, Anderson, Khait, Sunday, & Halmi, 1991).

Table 2-3 Heterocyclic Antidepressants and Their Uses

Trade Name	Generic Name	Other Uses
BuSpar	Buspirone	Sedative withdrawal*
		Premenstrual syndrome*
Desyrel	Trazodone	Cocaine withdrawal*
Floxyfral	Fluvoxamine	
Ludiomil	Maprotiline	Very similar to TCAs
Paxil	Paroxetine	
Prozac	Fluoxetine	Obesity*
		Bulimia*
		OCD*
Wellbutrin	Bupropion	
Zoloft	Sertraline	OCD*
*Unlabeled use		

The second generation AMs also produce their effects through the vehicle of raising levels of serotonin or up-regulating serotonin-2 receptors (5-HT2). Raising levels of 5-HT lowers depression in several important ways. Raising levels of 5-HT does the following:

- Inhibits stimulation of areas in the limbic system that produce emotional pain reactions
- Helps control obsessive rumination

- Aids in establishing proper sleep/awake cycles
- Suppresses long-term, low-level pain transmission
- Has important antianxiety effects
- Acts to regulate or modulate other neurotransmitters responsible for alertness (NE, for example). [Beasley, Masica, & Potvin, 1992; Delgado et al., 1991; Jonas & Schaumburg, 1991; Stahl, 1992]

CHARACTERISTICS OF SELECTED HETEROCYCLIC ANTIDEPRESSANTS

BuSpar (like the unreleased gepirone) is a selective serotonin (5-HT sub-1A) receptor agonist or enhancer. It is used primarily in the treatment of anxiety; however, research has also found that BuSpar, like other 5-HT partial agonist drugs, does have some antidepressant effects. These antianxiety and antidepressant properties are contradictory and are usually explained in the following way. As a partial agonist, buspirone or gepirone would compete with an oversupply of 5-HT, thus reducing its effects and acting as a functional antagonist. However, in depression (a deficiency of 5-HT) the drug's agonist properties would, first, allow the presynaptic membrane to replenish serotonin stores, and second, act as an agonist at the postsynaptic receptor in the condition of deficit 5-HT, which would cause a rise in activity and, thus, raise depression. Adjunctive use with other antidepressants is not fully researched (Napoliello & Domantay, 1991; Olin et al., 1993).

FLOXYFRAL (FLUVOXAMINE).   Not yet released for general use, fluvoxamine appears to be as effective as the TCAs. Its mode of action is the reduction of serotonin turnover. Like many of the heterocyclics, it appears to positively affect obsessive-compulsive syndromes, possibly through autoreceptor desensitization. Additional trials are required before it can be widely marketed. Like other AMs, fluvoxamine is likely to provoke mania in some bipolar clients (Olin et al., 1993).

PAXIL (PAROXETINE).   Paroxetine, one of the newer antidepressants on the market, was introduced in early 1993. Like sertraline and fluoxetine, it exerts its action by inhibiting serotonin reuptake, thereby increasing the amount of serotonin. Paroxetine can be given once daily, usually in the morning. The initial dose is 20mg per day and can be increased to 50mg daily. Similar to all antidepressants, the full therapeutic effect may be delayed. Side effects are relatively mild and are dose-related. Patients usually develop tolerance to its adverse effects (Olin et al., 1993).

PROZAC (FLUOXETINE).   Fluoxetine is now the most frequently prescribed antidepressant, with more than 800,000 prescriptions written each month (Jonas & Schaumburg, 1991). Research shows that fluoxetine has fewer side effects for most people than TCAs, producing a less "drugged" feeling. Fluoxetine accomplishes its antidepressant effect by raising levels of the neurotransmitter serotonin (5-HT) through the mechanism of decreasing its reuptake by the presynaptic neuron; that is, through downregulation of presynaptic inhibitory autoreceptors (Beasley et al., 1992). It appears to differentially affect 5-HT2 receptors believed to be particularly important in the regulation of mood.

Side effects and drug interactions. Fluoxetine has endured great controversy. Claims against fluoxetine based on anecdotal evidence have associated its use with acts of violence and suicide (Beasley et al., 1991). However, the FDA has ruled to keep fluoxetine on the market because its low risk of associated paradoxical effects appear no greater than risks associated with other AMs. The National Mental Health Association has maintained that fluoxetine is extremely useful in treating depression. Recommendations are to begin with a dose of 20mg in the morning. If no improvement is noticed within several weeks, the dose is increased. Full antidepressant effects may be delayed until four weeks. At the time of this writing, only two deaths from an overdose of fluoxetine have been reported; autopsies on both cases indicated that other drugs were involved. Finally, although drinking alcohol should be firmly discouraged since it is often addictive and certainly exacerbates depression, fluoxetine has very low levels of interaction with alcohol (Jonas & Schaumburg, 1991).

WELLBUTRIN (BUPROPION). Because of the possibility of seizures, alcohol consumption is ill-advised when taking bupropion. Levodopa, lithium, and fluoxetine should also be avoided. Motor coordination may be impaired with its use. Wellbutrin exerts its effects by inhibiting dopamine reuptake (Ferris, Cooper, & Maxwell, 1983), a mechanism similar to that of stimulant drugs (cocaine) and, secondarily, by inhibiting turnover (reuptake) of norepinephrine. Several of its metabolites also appear to have antidepressant properties (Goodnick, 1991). Bupropion's potential for abuse is unclear. It has been used in the treatment of cocaine abuse, Parkinson's disease, and chronic fatigue syndrome without significant adverse reactions (Goodnick, 1991).

ZOLOFT (SERTRALINE). Sertraline, which is similar to fluoxetine, was approved for marketing in December 1991. Antidepressant actions are due to the inhibition of 5-HT reuptake. Its effects may be delayed.

DEPRESSION IN THE ELDERLY

Age and depression are highly and positively correlated (Plotkin, Gerson, & Jarvik, 1987). This is particularly true when social attachments deteriorate among the aging (Mullins & Dugan, 1991). Age-related depressive effects include decreased metabolic activity, cerebral blood flow, oxygen metabolism, and neurotransmitter concentrations (Busse & Simpson, 1983; Yesavage, 1992). Although the elderly represent only 12 percent of the population, they account for 20 percent of suicides (6,000) each year (Yesavage, 1992).

Among this group, depression is often masked by or mistaken for physiological or other psychological problems. Physiological masks include loss of memory and concentration, gastrointestinal problems, poor overall health, arthritic changes, and heart disease (Yesavage, 1992), and other drug use (Crook, Kupfer, Hoch, & Reynolds, 1987). Masking psychological problems include anxiety, grief, insomnia, confusion, impulsivity, unwarranted anger, and apathy (Fredrick & Fredrick, 1985; Yesavage, 1992). Depressed geriatric clients usually do not have a long history of memory loss, disorientation, incontinence, neurological signs such as muscle weakness or **ataxia** (loss of coordination), or aphasia (loss of speech production facility or loss of social appropriateness) (Yesavage, 1992). Further, they are usually oriented, even though they may be too angry to answer questions, and their cognitive problems are erratic, rather than continuous.

All elderly clients need thorough assessment because of their heightened sensitivity to drugs and to social effects. The most effective forms of psychotherapy with the elderly emphasize re-engaging the client (and spouse or family) in activities that will increase cognitive, emotional, and social-behavioral awareness and that rely on social (or institutional) support to decrease negative rumination and isolation (Busse & Simpson, 1983; Mullins & Dugan, 1991; Mishara & Kastenbaum, 1980).

Yesavage (1992) points out, first, that if the client does not respond to psychotherapy he or she should certainly be referred for antidepressant therapy; second, he notes that the best antidepressant would be one that has few side effects, a short half-life, no active metabolites, and would induce few interactions with other drugs. Unfortunately, the tricyclic antidepressants do not fit this profile very well (Branconnier et al., 1983). But the heterocyclic AMs do fit this profile; sertraline (Zoloft), a serotonin reuptake inhibitor, has low anticholinergic effects, low lethality on overdose, low sedation, a moderately low half-life, does not potentiate alcohol, and produces few drug interactions (Olin et al., 1993). It should be remembered that sensitivity to AMs, especially amitriptyline, rises with age and that, therefore, smaller doses are more likely to be adequate for older clients. AMs are also more likely, even at low doses, to produce interactions with other medications older adults may be taking (Dawkins & Potter, 1991).

BIPOLAR AFFECTIVE DISORDER

Bipolar affective disorder (BAD) is commonly referred to as manic-depression. Criteria established by the DSM-IV (APA, 1994) state that an individual must have at least one episode of mania and one of depression to be diagnosed with BAD. An accurate diagnosis may be difficult because approximately 30 percent of all patients having a manic episode experience hallucinations or delusions, which makes it difficult to separate BAD from schizophrenia or other psychosis-inducing illness. Unfortunately, where symptoms of BAD are confused with features of schizophrenia, misdiagnosis can lead to administration of inappropriate drug therapy, often for long periods of time.

Somewhere between 0.4 and 1.2 percent of the general population is affected by BAD, with males and females being equally affected (Rosenbaum, 1988). For diagnostic purposes, bipolar disorders are divided by DSM-IV (APA, 1994) into four categories:

1. Mixed (currently alternating mania and depression)
2. Manic (not currently depressed)
3. Depressed (not currently manic)
4. Cyclothymic (presence for at least two years of numerous hypomanic episodes interspersed with episodes of depression that do not meet the criteria for major depressive episodes)

BAD includes rapid cyclers (those who move from depression to mania and back over a period as short as 24 hours) and those who cycle slowly, sometimes with only one manic episode each year.

ETIOLOGY

BAD results from a chemical imbalance in the brain, not from sociological factors. Positron emission tomography (PET) scans show remarkable differences in brain activity between the manic and depressive cycles. The manic, hyperexcited phase is apparently brought on by a lack of reuptake of excitatory neurotransmitter NE into the presynaptic membrane. The depressive phase is thought to be brought on by exhaustion of the production of excitatory neurotransmitters, by changes in responsiveness of the receptors for these neurotransmitters, or by hormonal changes that are triggered by hyperexcitability (Julien, 1992; Lickey & Gordon, 1983). Both abnormal neurotransmitter activity and receptor responsiveness are noted in patients with manic-depression. The occurrence of BAD is greatly influenced by genetics and, like unipolar depression, 60 to 80 percent of individuals with first-degree relatives who experience BAD will also experience some form of depressive syndrome (Restak, 1988). It is important for counselors to remember that clients' knowledge or intuitions about the very high incidence of genetic transmissibility may cause hopelessness and learned helplessness. This may occur even within high-risk offspring to whom the syndromes have apparently *not* been transferred.

TREATMENT

Lithium was first used for treatment of mania in the 1940s. Since that time, it has been established that manic-depression is effectively controlled by administration of lithium in approximately 80 percent of cases (Baldessarini, 1993). Many of those who do not do well on lithium alone can be treated successfully with a combination of lithium and carbamazepine (Tegretol) (Shukla & Cook, 1989). No studies support the effectiveness of psychotherapy alone for the treatment of BAD. Further, lithium has not been found to be effective with other forms of depression (Lickey & Gordon, 1983).

Psychotherapy is very useful, however, in treating the problems of living that often arise from BAD even when cyclic episodes are under relatively adequate control. Unfortunately, those who suffer from bipolar illness are poorly understood by the general public and, often, by their own families. Bipolar patients often have long histories of rejection, relationship difficulties, and issues of self-esteem and self-efficacy.

Many who suffer from bipolar disorder, especially those who are cyclothymic (cycles of **hypomania** and then mild to moderate depression), find it difficult to give up the highs, even though the lows are very painful. Cyclothymic individuals often discontinue usage of the drug because they no longer experience their lives as being creative, energetic, or fruitful, or because they feel overwhelmed by the drug's early side effects. Fortunately, most clients with bipolar disorder find that their creativity and energy are not diminished over the long run, even though their disorganization and depression are controlled by the lithium medication. During fully manic episodes, the client moves from feelings of extreme well-being, euphoria, control, and purpose, to feelings of being inspired, all encompassing, all knowing and omnipotent, while behaviorally growing more and more disorganized and impulsive. Particularly in the manic phase, but sometimes during depression, the patient may become psychotic, primarily delusional; hallucinations are not common. Men and women appear to react in much the same manner to lithium; however, current research reported by Dawkins and Potter (1991) indicates that malformations occurred in 11 percent of babies born to a sample of 225 women on lithium treatment.

REFERRAL

Manic clients or depressed clients having had a manic episode should be referred to a physician for psychiatric evaluation. Clients who appear cyclothymic but who are subclinical, should be monitored closely. It is unfortunate that when clients move into a hypomanic phase—or beyond it—it is often very difficult to get them into treatment because of their overwhelming feelings of well-being and power. Many clients in a severe manic phase must be mandated into a safe treatment setting. The counselor should be aware of the necessary protocol for civil commitment or confinement in the event that their client becomes psychotic. Individual treatment for bipolar disorder should include family education and therapy whenever possible. Family members often have issues with the client that need addressing and that have been suppressed because of the client's illness. Compliance or hospitalization will be facilitated if the counselor has a trusting relationship with, or at least a clear communication route to, the family or the significant other.

COMPLIANCE

Compliance issues found in all depressions are important in BAD. Compliance is complicated in BAD (a) by the client's desire for and sometimes dependence on the pleasurable, euphoric feelings that accompany the initial stages of mania, (b) by the impulsive nature of the manic phase of the disease, and (c) by the narrow therapeutic window within which lithium is effective. Often clients are in a hypomanic or depressed state (low lithium balance) or toxic state (high lithium balance) before they recognize it. If they go into a hypomanic state, clients are likely to discontinue their medication entirely because they feel so amazingly "well." As many therapists have discovered, helping a manic client recognize that medications are necessary cannot only be very difficult but very disconcerting as well due to the client's feelings of omniscience. Compliance is also complicated among BAD clients who are depressed because they may be agitated, hypervigilant, or frankly paranoid about their medication. In these situations, a liaison with the client's physician is very important. Liaison with the family of origin is important as well; however, this liaison should be developed only to the extent that the family is supportive and has a successful record of helping the client monitor behavioral difficulties. Otherwise, family therapy, not liaison, is called for.

PHARMACOKINETICS

Lithium, one of the basic elements of chemistry, is a positively charged ion. Neurons within the body react to lithium in a manner similar to sodium or potassium. Lithium is administered orally in a salt form and rapidly absorbed. Lithium is not protein bound, and it is not metabolized. About 95 percent of lithium is excreted unchanged in the urine. Passage of lithium across the blood-brain barrier (BBB) and placental barrier occurs easily and can produce **teratogenic effects** (developmental defects in utero) in infants. Because lithium is similar to sodium (found in table salt) in both size and electrical charge, the body's lithium level is influenced by the sodium level. Patients with high sodium levels excrete more lithium, while low sodium levels trigger the body to retain greater amounts of lithium. Thus, if clients lower their ordinary salt intake (through dieting, for example), more lithium will be retained in the body. Then, if they take in large amounts of table salt when they go off their diets, a toxic level of lithium will be reached in a very short time. Clients should have the relationship between lithium and table salt explained clearly and often. The activities that make clients' salt levels fluctuate (diet, exercise, and sweating) need to be fully discussed. Lithium's half-life is dependent on kidney functioning, with the average adult lithium half-life being 24 hours (Olin et al., 1993). There are a variety of trade names for lithium; among the most common are Eskalith, Lithane, Lithium Carbonate, Lithium Citrate, Lithobid, and Lithonate.

MECHANISM AND ACTIONS

The mechanisms of action for lithium's effects on both mania and depression are not fully understood. As stated above, lithium decreases mania by stabilizing the presynaptic membrane in such a way that 5-HT and NE can be reuptaken into the terminal vesicles. How this creates antidepressive effects is less clear. However, this may be accomplished by stabilizing the postsynaptic receptors so that NE can bind in a more effective way or by the effects on the endocrine system (Govoni & Hayes, 1985). Although lithium crosses the BBB quickly, the antimanic effect is delayed, usually for one to two weeks. During this delay period, antipsychotics (for example, phenothiazines such as Thorazine) may be used to control manic episodes.

LITHIUM'S SIDE EFFECTS AND TOXICITY

Lithium's side effects are dose-dependent, meaning larger lithium doses will produce more notable adverse effects. Lithium has a narrow therapeutic window with no great difference between effective and toxic doses. Lithium is monitored for the appearance of side effects along with careful observations of lithium blood levels (Schatzberg & Cole, 1986). It is not certain whether lithium causes kidney damage in otherwise healthy patients. However, if there is a personal or family history of kidney dysfunction, kidney function should be closely monitored. Finally, because it is teratogenic, lithium treatment should be avoided during pregnancy if at all possible. Other drugs should be substituted.

EARLY SIDE EFFECTS. Symptoms that often precede normal adjustment to lithium treatment are nausea, fine hand tremor, **polyuria** (increased urination) and **polydipsia** (increased thirst). These side effects usually subside within several weeks and are considered to be an inconvenience rather than a disabling condition.

EARLY WARNINGS OF MILD TOXICITY. Early warnings of toxicity include diarrhea, nausea, vomiting, sedation, lack of coordination, slurred speech, and increasing confusion. Reduction in lithium dosage is the recommended treatment in cases of mild toxicity. Severe toxicity can lead to seizures, coma, and death. Unfortunately, symptoms of toxicity are similar to early side effects. Lithium intake should be reduced and the client immediately referred back to his or her physician for consultation should there be doubts about toxic effects (Olin et al., 1993).

DOSAGE. Lithium dosage will vary depending on the phase of the illness and the side effects experienced by the patient. In the acute manic phase, the normal dose is 600mg three times per day or, if using a time-released drug form of lithium, 900mg twice a day. Lithium blood levels are checked twice weekly during the acute phase. Effective lithium blood levels are usually within 1–1.5meq/liter range. In the maintenance phase, weekly visits to the physician are recommended during the first month until the patient is stabilized. After stabilization on lithium, blood level range is 0.6–1.2meq/liter. Lithium doses in this phase will vary but are usually 300mg three or four times a day. Lithium levels should be monitored every two to three months (Olin et al., 1993).

Patients should be advised to take lithium immediately after meals or with food or milk to avoid stomach upset. It is also recommended that patients drink 8 to 12 glasses of water a day, maintain a salt-free diet, and avoid using diuretics, including coffee and alcohol (Olin et al., 1993). It is particularly important to note that many clients with bipolar illness have histories of self-medicating with alcohol and other substances that can enormously complicate drug treatment and psychotherapy. Therapists need to explore the client's alcohol and other drug use extensively as they assess the client's self-sufficiency.

ALTERNATE TREATMENTS FOR BAD

Even though lithium is the drug of choice for mania and bipolar disorder, there are instances when it cannot be used. Approximately 20 to 30 percent of patients with BAD are unresponsive to or do not tolerate lithium (Maxmen, 1991). When a patient cannot take lithium, the depression and mania are treated separately. Alternate treatments for mania include antipsychotics and antidepressants

Haloperidol (Haldol) or drugs in the phenothiazine class are also used for mania and are, sometimes, more effective in the treatment of severe mania. However, the side effects of antipsychotics are more troublesome. Additionally, the concomitant use of antipsychotics and lithium may increase the chance of precipitating the potentially fatal neuroleptic malignant syndrome (see Chapter 4).

Anticonvulsants are sometimes more effective than lithium in treating rapidly cycling patients. The benzodiazepine clonazepam (Klonopin), carbamazepine (Tegretol), and valproic acid (Depakene) have all been used as alternatives to lithium therapy. However, their effectiveness in treating the depressive phase of BAD is questionable (Maxmen, 1991).

CONCLUSION

The study of depression and bipolar disorder is proceeding rapidly from both etiological and treatment directions. Biochemists involved in developing and testing antidepressant and antimania drugs have helped treatment specialists provide better care; clinicians have supplied invaluable information to research and development specialists. Because combatting depression is financially rewarding, research has been hastened. However, the very success of AMs in relieving many of the symptoms—and, often, many of the underlying causal features of depression—has produced a backlash. This backlash has taken the form of media exposés of the overprescription of AMs or inadequate monitoring of long-term drug therapy. It is our hope that clients will be referred to physicians for screening for medication (a) only after an adequate regime of talk therapy has failed to provide needed relief, and (b) only if long-term use of the medication is closely monitored.

3

ANXIETY AND THE ANXIOLYTICS

SLEEP DISORDERS AND THE HYPNOTICS

This chapter provides an introduction to the underlying causes of anxiety, as well as the relationship between its etiology and its treatment. We also discuss the referral issues involved, such as the circumstances under which clients should be referred for screening for anxiolytics and when a client should not take anxiolytics. Later in the chapter, we cover the etiology and treatment of panic attacks. Finally, we discuss various sleep disorders and recommended treatments, including the use of hypnotic agents to treat some of these disorders.

ANXIETY

Psychology, from its earliest psychodynamic beginnings to modern existentialism, has viewed anxiety as the central dilemma of social existence. It is not surprising, therefore, that social anxiety is the most common form of psychological problem or that anxiety is the central concern of psychotherapy. Neither, then, should it be surprising that antianxiety drugs, also referred to as **anxiolytics** or **minor tranquilizers**, are the most widely used psychiatric medications. Seventy percent of all psychiatric medications prescribed are anxiolytics, and the majority of those are sedative-hypnotic benzodiazepines (BZDs). The high prescription rate for antianxiety agents (70 percent of which are prescribed for women) is probably not explained by reference to any single cause. Contributing factors are

41

the high levels of stress under which individuals (particularly women) live and work and the continued "medicalization" of anxiety. About 65 million prescriptions for BZD medications are written each year (Garvey, 1990). This is a staggering number given that anxiety is normal and necessary to protect us from risky or foolish behavior, that BZDs produce both physical and psychological dependence and are widely abused, and that BZDs are potentially fatal when taken in amounts over recommended doses or are combined with alcohol or other system depressing drugs that commonly produce additive or supra-additive effects.

When anxiolytics are prescribed without an adequate psychological assessment, the patient is put at risk in several ways. First, deeper personality problems underlying the anxious feelings may be further suppressed. At the same time, because BZDs loosen impulse control, underlying hostilities toward self or others may rise to the surface and be acted on explosively. For example, anxiety often masks depression. Depression coupled with low impulse control accounts for a majority of suicides. Second, because BZDs and barbiturates are dependency-producing or addicting, there is disagreement about whether they should be taken prophylactically for long periods of time. Third, physicians who are not in the mainstream of psychiatric services but who prescribe BZDs may not encourage patients to begin anxiety management psychotherapy (AMP). Fourth, like all sedative **hypnotics,** BZDs can loosen impulse control; patients without adequate drug education and adequate self-monitoring may impulsively take risks (take drugs they would ordinarily be too anxious to take, for example).

BZDs need careful controls (Tyrer & Seivewright, 1984). In our view (a view shared by many in the drug treatment field), BZDs should rarely be used for more than several weeks. Long-term BZD therapy should be considered only in the event that psychotherapy has clearly been shown to be unsuccessful.

DIAGNOSIS

The DSM-IV (APA, 1994) describes a wide range of anxiety disorders, including generalized anxiety disorder, simple phobia, social phobia, obsessive-compulsive disorder, posttraumatic stress disorder, panic disorders, and agoraphobia without history of panic disorders. All anxiety disorders commonly include motor tension, autonomic hyperactivity (shortness of breath, palpitations, sweating, dizziness), vigilance, and scanning. Each specific disorder includes further characteristic features. Individuals with anxiety disorders are often successful at controlling their anxiety by avoiding situations that trigger it or by self-medication with alcohol. Avoidance may lead to a constriction of interpersonal and economic circumstances. For example, people with social phobias may not be able to advance in their jobs if advancement requires making speeches, teaching, or giving presentations. Many anxious people medicate their problems with alcohol even though alcohol, because of rebound hyperexcitability, may exacerbate those problems. Unfortunately, like the other sedative-hypnotic drugs, alcohol can produce dependence and, for many, addiction.

Anxiety disorders may be divided into those that are spontaneous and thought to arise from genetic predisposition (generalized anxiety and obsessive-compulsive disorders, for example), those that arise through a conditioning experience (posttraumatic stress disorder (PTSD), for example), and signal anxieties that are thought to arise from unconscious conflicts. Each of these disorders can give rise to or be accompanied by panic attacks.

ETIOLOGY

Arousal elements in anxiety, normal or abnormal, are caused by either a decrease of an inhibitory neurotransmitter (GABA, for example) or an overabundance of an excitatory neurotransmitter (norepinephrine, for example) or both. Interpretation of an arousal state as anxiety, however, is dependent upon or mediated by culture-bound cognitions. Thus, what is happy excitement for one person may be anxiety for another, even though the physiological states are not distinguishably different. Very low levels of inhibitory neurotransmitters and very high levels of excitatory neurotransmitters are known to cause strokes, seizures, paranoia, and panic. Thus, abrupt discontinuation of a tranquilizing medication (inhibitory, sedative-hypnotic BZD, for example) and the subsequent rapid rise of excitation can cause the same symptoms as an overdose of a stimulant medication (adrenaline, for example). This state is called **rebound hyperexcitability.**

Panic states are caused by extreme reactivity of the centers in the brain that ordinarily alert the individual to impending danger. These centers, comprising the ascending reticular activating system (ARAS) of the brain, are rich in norepinephrine (NE). In the panic condition, these centers are bathed in NE, and the level of inhibitory neurotransmitter (GABA and serotonin 5-HT, for example) is insufficient to quiet the system (Julien, 1992).

Further, in areas of the brain concerned with sleep, feeding, and sexual activity (which are primarily rostral projections from the brain stem to the cerebral cortex, hippocampus, hypothalamus, and limbic system), 5-HT acts as an inhibitory neurotransmitter in opponent process with the excitatory neurotransmitter NE. Opponent process in this context implies acting in opposition to the excitatory effects exerted by NE. Thus, raising levels of 5-HT, as most second generation antidepressants do, down-regulates activity in these areas. Heterocyclic drugs known to raise 5-HT are fluoxetine (Prozac), sertraline (Zoloft), and fluvoxamine (Floxyfral). Both fluoxetine and sertraline also down-regulate sensitivity of NE receptors, which accounts for their ability to decrease depression without increasing mania as the tricyclics often do. One tricyclic antidepressant, clomipramine (Anafranil), is also thought to specifically raise levels of serotonin and is successfully used in treating obsessive-compulsive disorder, which appears to be related to abnormally low levels of serotonin.

Of particular importance is the regulation of proper levels of 5-HT in the brain's pontine raphe nuclei, a group of nerve cells that serves as a filtering system for incoming stimuli. 5-HT filters the flood of incoming information, letting through the most important and filtering out the less relevant. Interestingly, when **lysergic acid diethylamide (LSD)** competes with 5-HT at serotonin-2 receptors, it allows an unfiltered flood of sensory data that overloads the system and causes a wide range of cognitive and emotional distortions (Julien, 1992). These include, but are not limited to, feelings of unreality; novel cognitions, perceptions, and emotions; disorientation to time; and depersonalization or hyper-personalization. Further, many users experience sleeplessness, anxiety, paranoia, and panic. These last characteristics are caused by inadequate levels of 5-HT.

Confirmation of the inhibitory and regulatory functions of serotonin, and therefore the utility of the serotonin reuptake blocking antianxiety medications, comes from several divergent sources. Unfortunately, this picture is complicated by several factors. First, the final action of serotonin is not an inhibitory one in all areas of the brain. If serotonin acts to inhibit an area of the limbic system whose function is to suppress an emotion or behavior, it can be said to activate that emotion. In this case, 5-HT can act as an antidepressant in its final outcome. This is the case in its effects on depression through regulation of the sleep cycle. A major part of the utility of fluoxetine in lowering depression may well be in its regulation of sleep. Second, and less well understood, most neurotransmitters can be either excitatory or inhibitory depending on where their effects are measured. What is clearly inhibitory in one locus of the brain may well be excitatory in another.

In conclusion, we are discovering that low serotonin is responsible for a wide range of emotional disturbances that includes both depression and anxiety. Therefore, use of medications that enhance 5-HT are likely to rise. At present, 800,000 prescriptions are being written each month for Prozac alone. Zoloft, another heterocyclic antidepressant, is also rapidly gaining hold in the marketplace, particularly for geriatric depression and agitation, because it apparently has fewer side effects, has a rapid onset, and produces fewer interaction problems with other medications.

TREATMENT

Anxiety is often life-long unless treated because the predisposition to anxiety is genetically driven. Children with a first-degree family member suffering from anxiety will also suffer anxiety in approximately 50 percent of cases—even when they are not raised by their biological parents (Barlow, 1988). Second, learned anxiety generalizes. When anxiety is conditioned through a particular event (punishment, for example), the site of punishment and other conditions surrounding the punishment may be sufficient to evoke the anxiety over an extended period of time. Third, anticipation of panic is itself a potent causal agent of further anxiety. Fear reactions may be so aversive in and of themselves that anticipation of that fear may give rise to anticipatory anxiety that spirals upward in intensity. This anticipation is usually pushed forward by visualization of oneself in the panic condition. Fourth, unresolved psychological problems can produce anxiety.

Signal anxieties appear to arise from unconscious conflicts. In these cases, anxiety results from the activity of holding painful memories (sexual abuse, for example) under repression. From a psychodynamic perspective, the anxiety will only dissipate when these underlying issues have surfaced and been worked through. Our experience indicates that anxiety management programs that include progressive relaxation, desensitization through reciprocal inhibition, and cognitive restructuring are not usually successful over the long run with individuals whose anxiety stems from deeper, unresolved issues.

The prognosis for controlling anxiety through a combination of anxiolytics and psychotherapy is best if panic attacks, obsessive-compulsive features, major depressive episodes, and simple phobias are not central features of the condition. Stress-related and generalized anxieties have the best prognosis and yield to drug treatment in about 65 percent of cases without psychotherapy (Barlow & Cerny, 1988). Presumably, this rate would increase substantially when drugs and psychotherapy are utilized together.

Psychotherapy, primarily anxiety management programs (AMP), should be used in place of drug therapy wherever feasible for a number of reasons. First, because antianxiety medications are often addicting, they should not be taken for extended periods. Second, psychotherapy is useful in identifying and de-escalating anticipatory anxiety preparatory to panic incidents. Third, psychotherapy is less expensive and can support lifestyle changes that will reduce many of the health deficits that arise from anxiety and stress. And fourth, evaluation and treatment of underlying problems that may decrease drug treatment should be ongoing. See Box 3-1 for suggested uses of AMP and drug treatment.

Box 3-1   Anxiety Management Programs and Drug Treatment

Drug treatment without a formal anxiety management program is indicated if

- stressors leading to episodic anxiety are found to be of short duration and are situation limited,
- relaxation or other techniques are sufficient to trigger high levels of anxiety or panic episodes, or
- client has a history of lack of progress with at least two psychotherapy techniques, one of which is a structured anxiety management program.

AMP alone should be considered if

- client fails to respond to adequate trials of two anxiolytics or has an inability to tolerate medication side effects,
- client has only a partial response to adequate doses of anxiolytics,
- client fails or exhibits only a partial response to other less structured psychotherapeutic methods,
- stress or environmental triggers predominate, or
- cognitions are the most salient triggers of anxiety.

In addition, the following conditions should be met when using AMP alone:

- The client has no previous diagnosis of untreated affective (depressive) disorder.
- Panic attacks occur no more than once a year.
- Anxiety is not accompanied by mania or hypomania.
- The client is not presently dependent on or abusing alcohol or other drugs.

Sources: Barlow, 1988; Barlow & Cerny, 1988; Beck & Emery, 1985.

TREATMENT CONSIDERATIONS: THE CLIENT'S POINT OF VIEW

Individuals presenting for treatment of anxiety have often moved through a wide variety of precipitating events. Much anxiety is produced by both legal and illegal drugs, including the sedative hypnotics prescribed to help solve the anxiety problem in the first place. For many people, ordinary behaviors (speaking to a group of people, for example) may be interpreted as frightening, even though there is no clear threat. In these cases, the anticipatory anxiety becomes painful and embarrassing. Further, many activities thought necessary to survive in the modern world are, by the very nature of human evolutionary history, stressful. Human beings are not well designed for jobs that require constant vigilance or high levels of autonomic stimulation like that required of air traffic controllers or long-distance pilots. Finally, people who take stimulant drugs (cocaine, amphetamines, and even coffee) often experience debilitating panic attacks. Stimulant abusers who are having panic attacks often present themselves for treatment or referral to get prescriptions for tranquilizers so they can continue their drug abuse with less anxiety. Furthermore, a wide range of physical problems can cause anxiety, irritability, and agitation. Box 3-2 lists some of the more common conditions associated with panic and anxiety symptoms.

Most people discover at one time or another that alcohol is a powerful sedative hypnotic and anxiolytic, even if it is effective only over the short run. Unfortunately, like the majority of anxiolytic sedative hypnotics (benzodiazepines, for example), alcohol is addictive and causes rebound hyperexcitability when it is abruptly discontinued. Hyperexcitability due to abrupt discontinuation of long-term use of sedative hypnotics can cause strokes, seizures, feelings of depersonalization, anxiety, and panic attacks. Long-term withdrawal symptoms (in many cases longer than one year) make treatment more difficult and almost impossible if these effects are not taken into account and dealt with in therapy.

Box 3-2   Organic Conditions Associated with Panic and Anxiety Symptoms

- Asthmatic conditions
- Audiovestibular system disturbance
- Cardiac arrhythmias
- Cushing syndrome (increased cortisol output)
- Hyperthyroidism (excessive thyroid activity)
- Hyperventilation
- Hypoglycemia (low blood sugar)
- Hypoparathyroidism (deficient parathyroid activity)
- Mitral valve prolapse
- Pheochromocytoma (adrenal tumor)
- Postconcussion syndromes
- Temporal lobe epilepsy

Source: Szeinbach & Summers, 1992.

Long-term withdrawal symptoms include irritability, depression, craving, mood swings, and an exacerbation of the anxiety that the drugs were originally pre-scribed to control. When either alcohol or the BZDs are being abused for their euphoric effects, tolerance develops so that a higher and higher dose must be taken to produce the same effect. However, some studies have found that individuals without a history of alcohol or drug abuse who are prescribed BZDs usually do not increase their reported dose (Garvey, 1990; Roy-Byrne, 1992). Individuals who routinely use alcohol or short-acting BZDs are likely to go through *daily* rebound hyperexcitability.

Given these problems, the difficult withdrawal from prescription sedative hypnotics, and the high relapse back to BZDs for anxiety sufferers (Roy-Byrne, 1992), many counselors in the drug treatment field believe that these medications cause more problems than they cure.

THE THERAPIST'S POINT OF VIEW: THE MEDICATED CLIENT

Counselors are faced with several central concerns in treating anxious clients who are being medicated. First, there is evidence that having a client on an anxiolytic interferes with AMP by temporarily interrupting the connection be-tween the stimulus (for example, thoughts of speaking in public) and the re-sponse (anxiety) so that desensitization learning cannot occur (Sanderson & Wetzler, 1993). If no anxiety exists in the medicated client, no graded series of cognitive-emotional exercises to diminish the stress can take place. Reciprocal inhibition techniques do not work if there is no low-level stress to be inhibited; again, no learning takes place. Second, anxiety that arises from depression and that is treated with anxiolytics may exacerbate the depression and put the client at higher risk for suicide. This is true because anxiolytics are depressants on the one hand while their anxiolytic properties weaken impulse control on the other. Approximately 60 percent of all suicides are committed by depressed individuals under the influence of sedative-hypnotic drugs, usually alcohol (Julien, 1992).

Fortunately, unlike the barbiturate drugs, a dose of BZDs 60 times larger than a normal therapeutic dose is usually required for an adult male to commit suicide, assuming no other sedative hypnotic, including alcohol, has been consumed. Even in cases of large doses ingested, patients have rarely been successful in their attempts because suppression of breathing by BZDs is a lengthy and reversible process. However, alcohol and other depressants potentiate or geometrically increase the effects of the BZDs so that fewer are needed for suicide. Anxious patients who are also depressed should not be prescribed either barbiturates or synthetic barbiturates (methaqualone, glutethimide, or meprobamate), which are all life-threatening at less than 20 times the usual dose necessary to relieve anxiety or sleeplessness (Lickey & Gordon, 1983).

Anxiety management approaches are often sabotaged by clients dependent on sedative-hypnotic drugs because clients believe the drugs are crucial to their well being. The AMP tries to wean clients away from their drugs, and thus, client and program objectives are headed in opposite directions. To win, the client has only to discontinue treatment. A strong therapeutic alliance with the client and the client's physician is crucial for AMP to be effective. Often, alcohol or drug treatment is necessary before long-term sedativists can profit from AMP. Clients who are suspected of being dependent on sedative hypnotics, especially alcohol, should not be advised to discontinue their use abruptly. These clients need to be assessed for medical detoxification. This is especially true if the client is older or has had any symptoms of delirium tremens (DTs).

REFERRAL

Anxious clients should be referred for psychiatric screening for an anxiolytic under any of the following circumstances:

- The client is too anxious or paranoid to take advantage of a cognitive-behavioral anxiety management program.
- AMP or at least one other form of psychotherapy has been shown to be ineffective for this client at this time.
- There is a history of a first-degree family member whose similar anxiety responds favorably to anxiolytics and who has not formed a drug dependency.

AMP should be initiated in conjunction with the drug therapy as soon as the client's anxiety has been reduced to a level that makes AMP possible.

Barlow and Cerny (1988) and others (Barlow, 1988; Beck & Emery, 1985) have suggested that clients should be referred for psychiatric screening for both medical and psychiatric conditions under any of the following circumstances:

- Client has a history or family history of depression, including bipolar disorder.
- Client has a history or family history of psychosis.
- Client has a history or family history of endocrine or hormonal problems.
- Client has a history of brain injury or life-threatening injury.
- Client has a history of impulsive behavior, including life-threatening behavior.

Clients should not take anxiolytics, especially barbiturates and benzodiazepines, if they

- are not willing to consider psychotherapy as a co-therapy,
- are drinkers or illicit drug users,
- are using anxiolytics for more than three evenings in a row as a sleep medication (tolerance for their sleep-inducing effects develops quickly),
- have used anxiolytics for more than two months without a drug holiday lasting several weeks,
- are increasing their dosage beyond the ordinary range for nontolerant persons,
- are keeping large numbers of pills on hand, or
- are getting refills without consulting a physician.

ANTIANXIETY AGENTS

Antianxiety agents are more effective in anticipatory situations than in panic conditions. To avoid the lifelong use of antianxiety drugs, the source of the anxiety must be investigated and eliminated. Psychotherapy should be adjunct treatment for anxiety.

Other terms used to describe this collection of drugs are *minor tranquilizers* or *anxiolytics*. The term *minor tranquilizer* implies similarities to a group of drugs called major tranquilizers (antipsychotics); however, they are not the same. Use of the word *minor* to describe this group of addictive anxiolytics was a marketing strategy by the drug companies to smooth their introduction into the marketplace, a tactic obviously having enormous success. BZDs are an example of a popular class of minor tranquilizer; phenothiazines are an example of a class of major tranquilizers. Table 3-1 provides a comparison of the major actions for both groups of drugs and illustrates the differences.

Therapeutic Effects of Minor Tranquilizers: The onset of the desired effects of a minor tranquilizer can occur quickly, anywhere from 10 minutes to several hours, because BZDs are rapidly absorbed into the bloodstream (Ponterotto, 1985).

Dangers of Minor Tranquilizers: Tolerance, causing an increase in dosage, psychological dependence and addiction, and the potential to produce fetal abnormalities (Maxmen, 1991).

Side Effects of Minor Tranquilizers: Drowsiness, ataxia (lack of coordination) with high doses, slurred speech, and other signs of CNS depression are common side effects associated with antianxiety agents. Potential for successful suicide is moderate to low, unless this medication is used with other CNS depressants (Szeinbach & Summers, 1992).

Precautions: Abrupt discontinuation of antianxiety agents that have been used for a long time is ill-advised (Swonger & Matejski, 1991). Rebound hyperactivity may produce strokes, seizures, and panic states. This class of drugs should not be used for primary depression, primary psychosis (they may worsen psychotic agitation), or personality disorders (Olin et al., 1993).

Table 3-1 A Comparison of the Effects of Major and Minor Tranquilizers

Minor Tranquilizers (Benzodiazepines or BZDs)	*Major Tranquilizers (phenothiazines)*
Sedation	Sedation
Antianxiety	Extrapyramidal side effects
Central muscle relaxers	Neuroleptic state:
	Psychomotor slowing
	Emotional quieting (fewer
	hallucinations and delusions)
	Affective indifference
High addiction potential	No addiction potential

Source: Julien, 1992.

BENZODIAZEPINE ANTIANXIETY AGENTS

BZDs are often the treatment of choice for anxiety. BZDs do not cure anxiety but do reduce symptoms. Removal of all symptoms may not be desirable because anxiety is considered "both an emotion and an essential drive" and is primarily connected to "choice and uncertainty," both of which are necessary for functioning in the modern world (Leccese, 1991). Table 3-2 lists antianxiety drugs and their most common uses.

MISCELLANEOUS ANTIANXIETY AGENTS

Table 3-3 lists antianxiety agents other than BZD. It also lists daily dosages and the most common uses for each of these agents.

PANIC ATTACKS

A panic attack is a sudden episode of inappropriate intense fear, apprehension, or terror with multiple physiological symptoms. While only around 6 percent of the population experience multiple panic attacks yearly (Dugas, 1987), perhaps 34

Table 3-2   Specific Antianxiety Benzodiazepines and Their Uses

Trade Name	Generic Name	Daily Doses (Divided into 2–4 Doses)	Uses
Ativan	Lorazepam	1–10 mg	Anxiety associated with depression; preanesthetic sedative
Centrax	Praxepam	20–40 mg	Short-term for anxiety
Halcion	Triazolam	.125–.5 mg*	Primarily for sleep
Librium	Chlordiazepoxide	15–300 mg	Preoperative anxiety (given a few days before surgery); acute alcohol withdrawal
Paxipam	Halazepam	20–160 mg	Acute anxiety and sedation
Serax	Oxazepam	30–120 mg	Anxiety associated with depression
Tranxene	Clorazepate	15–60 mg	Adjunct to seizure treatment; acute alcohol withdrawal
Valium	Diazepam	2–40 mg	Acute alcohol withdrawal; adjunct muscle relaxer; adjunct anticonvulsant and preoperative; unlabeled uses—panic attacks
Xanax	Alprazolam	0.5–1.5 mg	Panic disorder; unlabeled uses—agoraphobia with social phobia; premenstrual syndrome

*One dose daily, taken at bedtime

Source: Olin et al., 1993.

Table 3-3   Antianxiety Agents Other than BZD

Trade Name	Generic Name	Daily Doses (Divided into 2–4 Doses)	Uses
Adapin, Sinequan	Doxepin[1]	25–400 mg	Anxiety; depression; somatic symptoms and concerns; insomnia; guilt; lack of energy; fear; apprehension; worry
Atarax, Vistaril	Hydroxyzine (antihistamine)		Itching; preanesthesia sedative; IM for acutely disturbed or hysterical patient or for withdrawal symptoms; as adjunctive medication to permit a reduction in dosages of narcotics
BuSpar[2]	Buspirone	15–30 mg	Unlabeled use—premenstrual syndrome; anxiolytic follow up after discontinunation of BZD or alcohol consumption
Equanil, Miltown	Meprobamate[3]	800–2400 mg	Similar to barbiturates; now used rarely for sleep and anxiety

[1]Doxepin is a tricyclic antidepressant with antianxiety action.
[2]BuSpar's mechanism of action is that of a selective (serotonin) 5-HT (1A) subreceptor agonist. Like other 5-HT agonists, BuSpar also has antidepressant effects. It has not been found effective in panic situations. BuSpar is less sedating than BZDs, but CNS effects may not be as predictable. No cross-tolerance with other CNS depressants (for example, BZDs or alcohol) appear to develop. Patients taking BuSpar do not develop drug dependency; therefore, it is safer than the BZDs. Optimum results are seen in three to four weeks.
[3]Has the highest suicide and addiction risk.

Sources: Maxmen, 1991; Napoliello & Domantay, 1991; Olin et al., 1993.

percent of the normal population experience one panic attack yearly (Barlow & Cerny, 1988). Thus, panic or anxiety attacks are very common. Their onset usually occurs in the late teens or mid-20s, and there is evidence for a genetic component for this disorder (Dugas, 1987).

ETIOLOGY

Spontaneous panic attacks (meaning no precipitating factor identified or both uncued and unexpected) are thought to have an organic basis. A neurochemical defect is suspected in the brain's locus ceruleus (an area of the brain stem). The locus ceruleus either amplifies or dampens incoming brain messages. In a panic attack, the incoming signal is misinterpreted or overinterpreted by the locus ceruleus, relaying panic messages to other areas of the brain (Charney, Heninger, & Breier, 1984).

Panic attacks can lead to agoraphobia. An individual having panic attacks may identify many causes for these unwanted episodes, creating anticipatory anxiety. Anticipatory anxiety can lead to extreme avoidance, the culmination of this avoidance may lead to an individual refusing to leave home. With this progression in mind, agoraphobia may be considered to be a more severe variant of panic disorder (Noyes et al., 1986).

TREATMENT

The most common mode of treatment for all anxiety problems is self-medication with alcohol. However, this method of treatment is not the most appropriate because excessive alcohol use can cause rebound panic attacks. Alcohol may worsen panic attacks because even mild alcohol withdrawal can intensify the problem (Woolf, 1983). In treating panic attacks, Dugas (1987) targets three groups of symptoms:

- *Emotional symptoms*, such as overwhelming fear or apprehension, fear of dying or going crazy
- *Physiological signs*, such as difficult breathing, increased heart rate, dizziness or nausea
- *Anticipatory anxiety*, which leads to more avoidance

Past research has shown that antianxiety agents do a poor job in eradicating panic attacks. This is true for a combination of reasons but primarily because a dose of BZDs capable of preventing uncued and unexpected panic attacks, is high enough to cause major side effects. Further, most uncued panic attacks, those not tied to specific external stimuli, occur before even the fast-acting BZDs can take effect. Cued and expected panic attacks, those caused by public speaking, for example, can be medicated successfully with a combination of a short-acting BZD and propranolol (Inderal), a beta-adrenergic blocker often prescribed to lower blood pressure, which helps control the rapid heartbeat and other physiological symptoms of norepinephrine-cued distress. Propranolol has been found to be effective in decreasing the cardiorespiratory symptoms of panic attacks while having no abuse potential.

In some cases the emotional symptoms and physiological signs are helped by using the tricyclic antidepressant imipramine (Tofranil) at 150–200 mg daily, or clomipramine (Anafranil), a serotonin reuptake inhibitor. Monoamine oxidase inhibitor (MAOI) antidepressants such as phenelzine (Nardil) are also used but require dietary restrictions. The second generation antidepressants, Prozac (fluoxetine) has also been found to have an inhibiting effect on both anxiety and panic and, particularly, on the anxiety dimensions of obsessive-compulsive disorder. Benzodiazepines (BZDs) often complement the effects of the antidepressants in treating panic attacks by helping to alleviate the anticipatory anxiety. One BZD, alprazolam (Xanax) at a dose of at least 4 mg daily is needed for successful treatment for the associated anxiety. However, chronic use of BZDs carries the risk of tolerance and dependence (Dugas, 1987; Roy-Byrne, 1992; Swonger & Matejski, 1991).

SLEEP DISORDERS

Sleep is a cyclic phenomenon. The various stages from wakefulness to deep sleep are recorded polygraphically with the assistance of an **electroencephalogram (EEG),** which measures brain waves (Moorcroft, 1989). The five stages are beta (awake and active), alpha (relaxed and sleepy), theta (asleep), delta (very deep sleep), and **rapid eye movement (REM) sleep,** during which the body is partially paralyzed and most dreaming occurs. Paradoxically, REM sleep is autonomically closest to wakefulness, and during the night we usually move through cycles of delta and REM sleep. Each sleep stage is characterized by different brain wave patterns. Sleep stages 1 through 4 are collectively referred to as *non–rapid eye movement* (non-REM). Some of stage 3 and most of stage 4 contain delta (slow) waves. **Delta waves** represent deep, restorative sleep. The brain's neurotransmitter serotonin plays an active role in non-REM sleep, while the neurotransmitter norepinephrine is vital to REM sleep and wakeful activity. REM sleep is characterized by regular fast eye movements, muscle paralysis, and dream activity. As the night progresses, REM sleep stages increase in length and become more intense psychologically and physiologically (Riley, 1985).

Sleep Deprivation

After a period of REM sleep deprivation, an individual will rebound by spending more sleep time in the REM stage. Effects of sleep deprivation are feelings of intense sleepiness, depressed mood, increased aggression, difficulty in maintaining prolonged concentration, perceptual distortions and, sometimes, mild hallucinations (Morris, Williams, & Lubin, 1960; Parkes, 1985). The DSM-IV categorizes sleep disorders into two main groups:

- **parasomnias**—an abnormal event during sleep
- **dyssomnias**—complaints of amount, quality, or timing of sleep [APA, 1994]

SLEEP DISORDERS AND RECOMMENDED TREATMENTS

Somnambulism (sleepwalking) is usually seen in children, who generally outgrow this sleep disorder. Approximately 10 to 20 percent of the population experience sleepwalking episodes. Sleepwalking occurs during delta wave sleep, and contrary to popular belief, it is not the "acting out" of dreams. Somnambulism is more likely to occur if an individual is tired, sleep deprived, under stress, or taking sleeping pills. Recommended treatment is to protect the sleepwalker by taking specific actions such as locking doors and giving the sleepwalker a first-floor bedroom (Moorcroft, 1989).

Night Terrors (sleep terror disorder or pavor nocturnus) are characterized by extreme vocalizations (usually occurring one-half to one hour after sleep onset), sweating, or fast heart rate (tachycardia). Night terrors are also a delta wave sleep phenomenon. Occurring mostly in children, night terrors are frequently outgrown. Benzodiazepines (BZDs), a chemical class of sedative-hypnotic drugs, suppress delta wave sleep. However, the risks associated with use of BZDs on the developing central nervous systems of children is unknown; therefore, use of BZDs in treating night terrors is not recommended (Hauri, 1985).

Nightmares (dream anxiety disorder) differ from night terrors in that nightmares are usually associated with elaborate and frightening content. In night terrors the individual is usually unable to recall a narrative. Additionally, nightmares occur during REM sleep rather than during non-REM sleep. Recommended treatment is that parents calm and reassure their child. For adults with frequent, disturbing nightmares, psychotherapy is suggested (Wincor, 1990).

Sleep Apnea (breathing-related sleep disorder) occurs mostly in men over 30 years old and is characterized by episodes of cessation in breathing producing many "mini-arousals" throughout the night. An individual suffering from sleep apnea may not be aware of the interruptions in normal breathing. Often the only complaints are headaches, irritability, or difficulty in daytime functioning. Two main causes for sleep apnea are (1) airway obstruction, as in enlarged tonsils, and (2) malfunctioning in the brain's respiratory centers. Treatment depends on etiology. A tonsillectomy or weight loss may eradicate the airway obstruction problem. In extreme (life-threatening) cases, a tracheostomy (airway vent in the throat) may be necessary. It is imperative to *avoid* all drugs with CNS depressant activity (including tranquilizers, hypnotics, sedatives, narcotics, and alcohol). Central nervous system–depressing agents are potentially lethal to an individual with sleep apnea. CNS depressants can interfere with the body's built-in mechanisms (mini-arousals) that function to block the prolonging of apnea episodes (Wincor, 1990).

Narcolepsy is characterized by uncontrolled sleep attacks of short duration. The most common features associated with narcolepsy include the following:

- Excessive daytime sleepiness
- Falling asleep at inopportune moments
- Cataplexy, a brief episode of muscle weakness that can result from experiencing strong emotions such as laughter or anger
- Sleep paralysis, an inhibition of musculature without unconsciousness (although seemingly awake, the individual is unable to move)
- Hypnogogic hallucinations, REM dreams that occur during wakeful sleep paralysis [APA, 1994]

However, the main symptom of narcolepsy is sleep attacks that last from two to five minutes.

Onset for narcolepsy occurs in adolescence, and there is evidence for a genetic basis for this disorder. Narcolepsy is thought to be caused by inappropriate neural mechanisms that produce REM sleep (Carlson, 1991). Nonpharmacologic treatment is to educate the family about narcolepsy, stressing that an individual suffering from narcolepsy is not lazy or unmotivated. Daytime naps, lasting 15 to 20 minutes, may be helpful.

CNS stimulants are used for daytime sleepiness. Because of problems with abuse and dependence when using drugs in the amphetamine class of CNS stimulants, other (often similar) types of stimulants are usually used to treat narcolepsy. Two such drugs are methylphenidate (Ritalin), which is also a frequently abused drug, and pemoline (Cylert) (Wincor, 1990).

Bruxism (teeth grinding) occurs mostly in children. As many as 15 percent of children may grind their teeth while sleeping. In some children, teeth grinding is only temporary, while in others, it may be more of a problem. In some instances, a dentist is consulted for treatment. Teeth grinding has not been clearly associated with psychological problems (Moorcroft, 1989).

Insomnia is associated with a perceived decrease in the quality or quantity of sleep that affects daytime functioning. Ninety-five percent of all adults experience insomnia at least once in their lives. Diagnosis of insomnia is subjectively determined by the individual. Many sleep difficulties are secondary to, or a symptom of, physical or mental problems such as pain, thyroid problems, worry, excitement, acute psychosis, mania or depression, sleep apnea, stimulant drugs, drug dependence, or drug withdrawal. Other reasons for insomnia can be disruption in circadian rhythms or environmental changes. Not much is known about the neurochemical basis for insomnia (Wincor, 1990).

Treatment of insomnia depends on the type of insomnia. Assessing the sleep pattern is important in formulating an accurate diagnosis and selecting appropriate treatment. There is no ideal hypnotic drug or agent that induces sleep. Every marketed hypnotic has at least one of the following drawbacks:

- The individual is unable to maintain sleep for the expected duration.
- The individual is able to maintain sleep throughout the night but suffers a morning hangover effect.
- Problems associated with dependence and tolerance and with abrupt withdrawal of a hypnotic agent produces rebound insomnia.

Hypnotics should not be used in chronic insomnia. The only exception to this rule is a condition called *nocturnal myoclonus* wherein frequent muscle jerks produce "mini-arousals" during sleep (Wincor, 1990).

CLASSES OF HYPNOTIC AGENTS

Hypnotics produce a state of CNS depression resembling normal sleep. Utilizing smaller doses of hypnotic agents causes a state of drowsiness. When used in this manner, these agents are called *sedatives*. Progressive dose-related effects of hypnotics or sedatives are clear (Julien, 1992):

antianxiety $\longrightarrow$ sedation $\longrightarrow$ hypnosis $\longrightarrow$ general $\longrightarrow$ coma $\longrightarrow$ death
(sleep)   anesthesia

Most hypnotics are habit forming; therefore short-term use (seven days) is recommended. One CNS depressant can be potentiated by other CNS depressants (alcohol or another hypnotic drug). Ingesting various CNS depressants together can be lethal!

BARBITURATES. Barbiturates are a class of CNS depressant drugs that were frequently prescribed as sedatives. Barbiturates are not prescribed as often today because they

- have a narrow margin of safety,
- have a moderately high abuse potential,
- produce many drug interactions by induction of liver enzymes, and
- suppress both delta wave sleep and REM sleep.

After use over 14 consecutive nights, barbiturates lose their sleep-inducing efficacy unless a higher dose is taken. Barbiturates exert their effect by interrupting impulses in the brain's reticular activating system (RAS), which is responsible for alertness and attention (Olin et al., 1993). The most common barbiturates are listed in Table 3-4.

BENZODIAZEPINES (BZDs). BZDs are effective hypnotics. Compared to the barbiturates, BZDs are somewhat less likely to produce tolerance and physical dependence; however, tolerance, dependence, and addiction do develop, and the onset of dependence is often insidious. The client takes the medication to help with a light to moderate insomnia; however, if the drug is discontinued after several weeks of use, the client will probably have severe insomnia for several evenings. Thus, the drug both cures and causes sleep problems. Fortunately, most clients who abandon use of the drug do finally sleep.

These agents are usually not lethal unless taken in relatively large doses (great difference exists between toxic and therapeutic doses). Geriatric doses should be reduced from normal adult doses (Maxmen, 1991).

Table 3-4 Common Barbiturates

Trade Name	Generic Name
Amytal	Amobarbital
Butisol	Butabarbital
Luminal	Phenobarbital
Mebaral	Mephobarbital
Nembutal	Pentobarbital
Seconal	Secobarbital

Source: Olin et al., 1993.

Mechanism of Action: BZDs act on the GABA (an important inhibitory CNS neurotransmitter) receptor complex by enhancing GABA's inhibitory (sedative) activity. BZDs usually decrease the period from retiring to sleep onset (latency) and decrease the number of awakenings. REM sleep is shortened by BZDs, and most BZDs suppress delta sleep (Wincor, 1990). Some common BZDs are listed in Table 3-5. Drowsiness, ataxia (defective muscular coordination), syncope (fainting), paradoxical excitement, rash, nausea, and altered libido are possible side effects of BZDs (Olin et al., 1993).

Halcion, a triazolam, is used widely because it has the least effect on delta sleep and is least likely to produce morning hangover. However, it is criticized for producing CNS problems: amnesia, anxiety, delusions, and hostility. Also, the unexpected effects it can produce (usually the drugs disinhibiting effects on impulse control) are often attributed to the individual instead of to the drug (Olin et al., 1993). Arguments about these effects and the client's legal responsibility for them have spawned a variety of lawsuits. Halcion is more helpful in assisting an individual with falling asleep than it is in sustaining a sleep state (Swonger & Matejski, 1991).

Another group of hypnotic agents includes the *antihistamine hypnotics*. A useful side effect of some antihistamines is sedation. Because there is little physiological addiction potential, antihistamines are considered safe hypnotics. It should be remembered, however, that discontinuation of antihistamines after a long period of use will probably result in poor sleep for several nights until the body adjusts to the lack of drug in the system. The most popular antihistamine hypnotic is Benadryl. The adult dose as a sleep aid is 50 mg at bedtime. Patients subjectively report that the effect of Benadryl (50 mg) is equivalent to phenobarbital (60 mg). Increasing the dose of Benadryl does not increase its hypnotic effect; it only increases the anticholinergic effects.

In addition to the classes of hypnotics we have discussed here, there are a number of miscellaneous hypnotics to consider. These are listed in Table 3-6. All these agents are DEA controlled substances.

Table 3-5   Benzodiazepines (BZDs)

Trade Name	Generic Name
Dalmane	Flurazepam
Doral	Quazepam
Halcion	Triazolam
ProSom	Estazolam
Restoril	Temazepam

Table 3-6   Miscellaneous Hypnotic Agents

Trade Name	Generic Name
Doriden	Glutethimide
Noctec	Chloral hydrate
Noludar	Methyprylon
Paral	Paraldehyde
Placidyl	Ethchlorvynol

Source: Olin et al., 1993.

4

PSYCHOSIS AND THE ANTIPSYCHOTICS

The term *psychosis* was once used to describe any mental disorder but now represents a collection of mental disorders manifested by inabilities in perceiving and testing reality and in communicating effectively with others to the extent that the individual cannot meet everyday demands (Thomas, 1985). Psychotic behavior that follows from the mental disorder is often active but seemingly purposeless, inappropriate, abnormal, and sometimes threatening if challenged.

Chronic psychotic states can be subdivided into several major domains, that may not be mutually exclusive etiologically. These subdivisions are:

- *organic brain syndromes,* which represent a loss or alteration in nerve cell functioning that can occur with dementia (including Alzheimer's, multiple sclerosis, autism, and AIDS) and drug intoxications;
- *affective disorders,* including manic psychosis or depressive psychosis;
- *schizophrenia;* and
- *schizoaffective disorders.* [Andreasen, 1989; Julien, 1992]

Brief or transient psychoses, typical in delirium and substance abuse, are diagnostic in schizophreniform disorders and are not uncommon features in borderline and schizotypal personality disorders.

It is commonly held that various clinical manifestations of psychosis share some physiological pathways and not others. Whether schizoaffective disorder is to be classified as a subcategory of schizophrenia or as an affective disorder or as a separate, independent process is not at all clear. Even though there is no consensus, treatment and research data appear to indicate that schizoaffective disorder should be included in the affective area (Silverstone, 1989). Support for this view derives from findings that clients with schizoaffective disorders, like bipolars, tend to respond better to lithium treatment and that schizoaffective lithium nonresponders tend to respond better to carbamazepine (CBZ, Tegretol), an anticonvulsant tricyclic, than they do to typical schizophrenia drugs (neuroleptics) such as the phenothiazines or haloperidol (Brown & Herz, 1989; Okuma, 1989).

Sensitivity to neuroleptics has been proposed as a possible diagnostic criterion for schizophrenia, whereas nonsensitivity indicates schizoaffective disorder or some other disorder (Brown & Herz, 1989). There have also been conflicting findings in attempts to establish the degree to which positive (hallucinatory) and negative (depressive) symptoms in this family of psychotic disorders are diagnostic. Even though depression is typically seen in schizophrenia and is frequently a side effect of neuroleptic drug treatment, symptoms of schizophrenia do not remit when depression remits (Silverstone, 1989). Further, evidence from family genetic studies indicates a close etiological connection between schizophrenia and schizotypal and paranoid disorders, and less connection between schizotypal and affective disorders (Andreasen, 1989; Baron et al., 1985).

Even though it is quite possible that neuroleptic resistant clients do not have schizophrenia, many are simply given higher doses of neuroleptics to capitalize on the general tranquilizing effects of the drugs rather than being taken off the drugs completely while a reanalysis of the problem is attempted (Brown & Herz, 1989). Treatment implications for the psychotic and nonpsychotic schizophrenia spectrum disorders and affective disorders are presented in Table 4-1.

Table 4-1 Treatment Recommendations for Psychotic and Nonpsychotic Disorders

Disorder	Recommended Treatment
Psychotic Disorders	
Schizophrenia	Neuroleptics
Affective disorders (manic and depressive psychosis)	Lithium, Tegretol, antidepressants
Schizoaffective disorder	Lithium, Tegretol, antidepressants
Nonpsychotic Disorders	
Nonpsychotic schizophrenia spectrum disorder	Outpatient psychotherapy; usually not medicated
Schizotypal p.d.	
Schizoid p.d.	
Paranoid p.d.	
Nonpsychotic affective spectrum disorder	Outpatient psychotherapy; usually not medicated
Borderline p.d.	
Cyclothymic	
Dysthymic (antidepressant)	

Source: Andreasen, 1989.

Antipsychotic medications are appropriate when any of these symptoms are present:

- Schizophrenia
- Mania
- Psychosis
- Acute agitation
- Withdrawal hallucinosis [Olin et al., 1993]

Some antipsychotics can cause useful side effects such as sedation, decreased anxiety, and mood elevation. However, if the patient's primary problem is insomnia, anxiety, or depression, antipsychotics should not be prescribed.

SCHIZOPHRENIA

Approximately 1 percent of the world's population suffers from schizophrenia (APA, 1994) and about half of the 175,000 patients in U.S. mental institutions have diagnoses of schizophrenia. Schizophrenia is a form of psychosis that apparently affects both sexes and all races equally. Early age of onset has been found to be an unfavorable prognostic feature in the illness. Mortality of victims is about twice the rate for individuals without schizophrenia (Allebeck, 1989). Between 15 percent and 50 percent of those with schizophrenia experience depression both prodromally to acute exacerbations of the psychosis (prior to onset) and after recovery (Heinrichs & Carpenter, 1985; Loebel et al., 1992; Marder et al., 1991; Siris et al., 1991). Thus, depression is a common cause of relapse into primary symptoms as well as a common result. Individuals with schizophrenia account for 500,000 hospitalizations each year (Bellack, 1989), most of which are in local community hospitals today rather than in mental institutions. Of the 3 million homeless, approximately half are chronically mentally ill, and many have schizophrenia and cannot manage their own money or their own care.

Schizophrenia is a difficult illness to control for many reasons. More than 20 percent of those with schizophrenia do not respond to antipsychotic medications, 30 to 50 percent refuse to take them for a variety of reasons, 20 to 30 percent relapse chronically even though they do comply with medical treatment, and approximately 30 percent experience significant, sometimes debilitating, side effects from the drugs (Bellack, 1989).

DIAGNOSIS OF SCHIZOPHRENIA

Schizophrenia is distinguished in DSM-IV (APA, 1994) by the following characteristics: (a) multiple psychiatric processes, (b) deterioration of functioning, (c) over six months in duration, (d) not due to affective disorder, and (e) includes delusions, hallucinations, and thought disturbances. DSM-IV divides schizophrenia into five general subtypes:

- *Catatonic,* marked by decreased reactivity, posturing, or purposeless activity
- *Disorganized,* marked by incoherent or incongruous affect without systematic delusions
- *Paranoid,* marked by systematic delusions
- *Residual,* marked by emotional blunting and loose association without persistent delusions or hallucinations
- *Undifferentiated,* not classifiable but clear hallucinations or delusions are present.

Another way to characterize the disease of schizophrenia is by globally categorizing symptoms into two groups:

Positive symptoms include *thought disorder,* evidenced by irrational, disorganized thinking; *delusions,* beliefs that are contrary to facts; and *hallucinations,* wherein an individual perceives something, usually auditory, that is not present. These symptoms usually ameliorate with neuroleptic treatment.

Negative symptoms occur in the absence of normal behaviors, and include flattened emotional response, poverty of speech, lack of initiative, and persistent inability to experience pleasure. This constellation of symptoms is also seen in individuals who have endured damage to the frontal lobe of the brain (Price & Lynn, 1986) and are resistant to neuroleptic treatment.

This dichotomy in symptom categorization suggests that different biochemical and neurological disorders may result in schizophrenia. However, most individuals with schizophrenia have a combination of positive and negative symptoms. Positive symptoms are usually alleviated by drug treatment, which decreases action at dopamine-2 receptors. Effects of this drug treatment tend to confirm that the positive symptoms are due to overactivity at dopamine-2 receptors (Price & Lynn, 1986).

DOPAMINE HYPOTHESIS

The **dopamine hypothesis** of the cause of schizophrenia or psychoses states that the positive signs of schizophrenia are due to overactivity of dopamine in the brain's mesolimbic system (Leccese, 1991). Evidence in favor of the dopamine hypothesis relates to the treatment of Parkinson's disease. In Parkinson's, dopaminergic neurons in the brain's substantia nigra are affected. Exogenous dopamine, given in the form of L-dopa, is administered to increase CNS dopamine activity. Although the exogenous dopamine may improve Parkinson symptoms, an unwanted side effect that sometimes develops with the use of L-dopa is schizophrenia-like behavior (Olin et al., 1993). Additionally, other drugs that increase the availability of CNS dopamine are also known to produce positive symptoms of schizophrenia (for example, the psychotomimetic agents cocaine and amphetamine). Finally, lysergic acid diethylamide (LSD) and phencyclidine (PCP) are both known psychotomimetics, and their use is often associated with exacerbations of schizophrenia.

TREATMENT OF SCHIZOPHRENIA

Like many of the major psychiatric illnesses, a **stress-diathesis model** (stress and underlying biological factors) has been proposed for psychotic relapses in schizophrenia. Even though it is clear that schizophrenia is caused by organic factors that necessitate lifelong adaptation, the chronicity or life history of the disease for each victim is greatly affected by stressors from the external environment. Lack of a stable home, family support, and worthwhile community involvement are examples of external stressors. At the same time, psychological resilience is influenced by external factors such as continuing education, counseling, and crisis intervention and can negate some stressors.

The instability of mood, disorganization in thought processes, and eccentricities of behavior among those with schizophrenia often cause them to feel socially inadequate, particularly in their family environment if family members are vigilant and intrusive (even when clients are in remission). This social distress adds to normal life stress, and the cumulative burden leads to psychological consequences, including low self-esteem and self-efficacy, social withdrawal, loneliness, boredom, and affective difficulties such as depression and anxiety.

Stress, depression, and anxiety are sufficient to cause an exacerbation or relapse of psychotic symptoms. Continued stress leads to chronicity. Chronicity exacerbates both positive and negative symptoms of the illness. And failure to manage symptoms effectively continues the cycle of rejection, relapse, and acting out.

RELAPSE. Contemporary therapy for those with schizophrenia emphasizes the role for neuroleptic drugs, the family, the community, and the individual in modifying the stress conditions that lead to relapse (Kane, 1989). Conditions that should alert counselors to a probability of relapse are

- increases in either positive or negative symptoms (20 to 50 percent experience depression prior to exacerbations),
- major stressors (including changes in living or job situation, familial intrusions or losses, changes in medications—compliance failure or reduction of dose, change in physician or therapist),
- use of alcohol or illicit drugs,
- physiological problems,
- problems with the legal system (20 to 30 percent have been incarcerated),
- changes in global assessment of functioning (GAF) as defined in the DSM-IV, or
- denial that the underlying illness is still present. [Kane, 1989; Marder et al., 1991]

Heinrichs and Carpenter (1985) provide the following list of late-prodromal symptoms and their relative frequency in relapse (decompensation) of 47 patients with schizophrenia: hallucinations (53 percent), suspiciousness (43 percent), change in sleep (43 percent), anxiety (38 percent), cognitive inefficiency (26 percent), anger/hostility (23 percent), somatic symptoms or delusions (21 percent), thought disorder (17 percent), disruptive inappropriate behavior (17 percent), and depression (17 percent). Finally, Marder et al. (1991) found that even relatively small changes in emotional-behavioral signs and symptoms in maintenance treatment for schizophrenia may be clinically meaningful.

GENDER DIFFERENCES. Interestingly, researchers have found that when confounding factors of age and marital status are controlled for, women with schizophrenia show a better course of hospital treatment, experience shorter hospitalization, and survive longer in the community after their first hospital admission than do men (Angermeyer, Kuhn, & Goldstein, 1990). Moreover, Angermeyer et al. (1990) found further support that men are hospitalized earlier than women and that the onset of their disorder is earlier. Thus, for reasons that are still not clear but that may relate to the prophylactic effects of higher estrogen levels, the course of schizophrenia is milder and social adaptation is better among women. Further, more women were involved in parenting their children, were more likely to be heterosexually active, and were more likely to be living with a partner of the opposite sex (Test, Burke, & Wallisch, 1990). However, this significant positive difference should not mislead therapists to believe that the course for any given individual female client will be better. Unfortunately, as women age, their relapse histories tend to look more and more like those of their male counterparts (Angermeyer et al., 1990).

CHILDREN. Few studies of the efficacy of antipsychotics in the treatment of psychoses among children have been undertaken (Gadow, 1992). One double-blind placebo-controlled study reported in Spencer et al. (1992) showed that haloperidol (Haldol) and loxapine (Loxitane) were superior to a placebo in controlling psychotic symptoms in children with schizophrenia. Spencer et al. (1992) found that haloperidol was effective enough and had limited enough side effects among a small group of hospitalized children with schizophrenia that they were able to continue on the medication after discharge. Side effects, including akathisia, neuroleptic malignant syndrome, and tardive dyskinesia are more likely among children with developmental disabilities than among other psychotic children. Even with proper dosage, neuroleptics are known to reach toxic levels quickly in children and to induce a variety of affective and behavioral problems (Gadow, 1992). Thus, their use should always be closely monitored by a professional who specializes in child psychiatry.

DEPRESSION IN SCHIZOPHRENIA. Because anxiety and depression are of particular importance to counselors who work with clients with schizophrenia, the following guidelines suggested by Johnson (1989) are presented to increase a practical understanding and approach to the relationship between psychosis and depression.

1. Overall, one-third of depressions among psychotics who are not having psychotic symptoms remit within two months without any change in treatment. The proportion is higher during the postpsychotic period.

2. The emergence of new depressive symptoms during remission of psychosis, particularly after an interval of one year, indicates incipient relapse.
3. Approximately 10 to 15 percent of depressed clients on maintenance neuroleptics are suffering from akinetic syndrome (muscular movement disorder), which responds to anticholinergic medication.
4. Pharmacogenic (drug-induced) depression must be considered. Dose reduction or change in drug must be considered.
5. Because tricyclic antidepressants can cause deterioration in those with schizophrenia, they should be used cautiously and closely monitored. Research is lacking in this area.
6. Clinical research into the uses of lithium present conflicting results; however, a therapeutic trial with patients with recurrent depressions may be useful. This is especially true if features of mania are present.
7. Minor tranquilizers given for agitation accompanying depression may cause the underlying psychosis to arise.

PSYCHOTHERAPY. As well as playing active roles in the emergency mental health networks in their communities, counselors in community mental health centers, medical settings, and private practice routinely play an important part in reinforcing the adaptation of clients with schizophrenia through consultation, psychotherapy, education, and referral. An understanding of the disease process itself as well as the neuroleptic medications for schizophrenia (and those used in conjunction to treat the affective components—anxiolytics and antidepressants) is crucial in facilitating clients' adaptive processes. As Coursey (1989) has said of this group, "They desperately need to understand what causes their disability and what does not, what intensifies their symptoms, and what their prognosis might be" (p. 350). Further, Coursey identified three important domains open to psychotherapy. First, psychological issues raised by the disorder that disturb core psychological functions (identity and efficacy for example). Second, those illness-related problems that the client can learn to self-manage. And third, those human problems that are not specific to schizophrenia but that require special attention because of the client's condition.

Although counselors, especially those who work with the chronically mentally ill, routinely take a case management approach, Coursey (1989) reasonably argues that counselors should use counseling skills rather than rely primarily on social work case management skills. In the same way that counseling the dying is not to prevent death but to help clients come to terms with death as human beings, the primary focus of psychotherapy among those with schizophrenia is not (as important as it is) to prevent relapse. Rather, counseling is meant to help the client come to terms with the life experience and meaning of the disease. While Coursey's view is well taken, it is important to note that psychotherapy cannot take place while clients are decompensating. Therefore, counselors must take a multifaceted approach in working with clients with schizophrenia.

It is also important that counselors realize, contrary to the way many research projects are framed, that medications and psychotherapy are not competitive but complementary. Complementarity in the relationship between psychotherapy and drug treatment is particularly important in working with individuals with schizophrenia, for whom prophylactic drug use is so pervasive and where the side effects of these drugs can be so profound and permanent. Fortunately for clients who are refractory to drug treatment, cognitive-behavioral and psychosocial strategies exist that are very successful in supporting remission (Brenner et al., 1990).

ANTIPSYCHOTIC DRUG ACTION

Terms used to describe the general category of antipsychotic drugs include **major tranquilizers**, **neuroleptics**, antischizophrenics, psychostatics, and **psychotropics**. Today, the term *neuroleptic* is principally used to indicate the phenothiazine drugs and Haldol that are used to treat the positive symptoms of schizophrenia such as psychoses. The antipsychotics block dopamine receptors in the brain, thereby preventing dopamine from exerting its maximum effect. Also, it is speculated that other neurotransmitters, such as glutamate, may be involved (Carlson, 1991).

THERAPEUTIC EFFECTS

Antipsychotics induce in schizophrenia what is called a **neuroleptic state** that is characterized by

> *psychomotor slowing* (decreased agitation, aggression, and impulsiveness),
> *emotional quieting* (decreased hallucinations and delusions), and
> *affective indifference* (not as concerned with external environment and not as
>   easily aroused).

Symptoms likely to improve are combativeness, tension, hyperactivity, hostility, and delusions. Symptoms that are not likely to improve are insight, judgment, and memory. Antipsychotics will help normalize sleep problems associated with many of the psychoses (Baldessarini, 1993). However, when administered to normal or asymptomatic individuals, antipsychotics may cause dysphoric or unpleasant effects (Julien, 1992). Consistent with the differences in chemical structure within the broad grouping of antipsychotics, these agents also differ in potencies and side effects (Ponterotto, 1985). The best prognosis for a patient taking antipsychotics is given to an individual with an acute psychotic episode who has a history of a healthy personality (Baldessarini, 1993) and a relatively short history of prodromal psychotic symptoms (Loebel et al., 1992).

SIDE EFFECTS

It usually takes two or more weeks for the drug's desired effect to occur, but side effects are often noticed sooner. Individuals taking antipsychotics must be warned about the delay of therapeutic effects. Adverse effects of antipsychotics are listed in Box 4-1.

Extrapyramidal side effects are explained in detail in the list that follows.

Parkinsonian symptoms are marked by rigidity and limited movement and are evidenced by **akinesia** (complete or partial loss of muscle movement), muscle rigidity, shuffling gait, drooling, mask-like facial expression, and tremor of extremities, especially the hands.

Dystonic reactions are involuntary and inappropriate postures and are evidenced by oculogyric crisis (fixed upward stare), torticollis (unilateral spasm of neck muscles), opisthotonos (arched back), and trismus, laryngospasm (spasm of muscles in jaw or throat).

Akathisia manifest as a compulsion to move, and an individual is in constant motion, exhibiting motor restlessness, an inability to sit or stand still, or rocking and shifting weight while standing.

Dyskinesia is inappropriate motor movement appearing early in treatment, and is evidenced by rhythmic clonic musculature contractions such as spasms, tics, and involuntary muscle movements.

Tardive dyskinesia is manifested by a rhythmical, involuntary movement of tongue, lips, or jaw, choreiform movements of extremities (jerky, purposeless movements), or athetoid movements of extremities (writhing, worm-like movements). [Thomas, 1985; Olin et al., 1993]

Box 4-1   Adverse Effects of Antipsychotics

Extrapyramidal Effects
Parkinsonian symptoms
Dystonic reactions
Akathisia
Dyskinesia
Tardive dyskinesia

Anticholinergic Effects
Dry mouth
Constipation
Blurred near vision
Urinary retention
Delayed ejaculation

CNS Effects
Sedation
Toxic psychosis
Seizures

Cardiovascular Effects
Orthostatic hypotension
EKG changes

Endocrine Effects
Amenorrhea (halt in menstruation)
Galactorrhea (breast milk production)
Gynecomastia (breast development)
Weight gain

Pigmentation Effects
Corneal, lenticular
Retinopathy
Skin

Allergic Effects
Hematologic
Skin
Hepatic

Source: Olin et al., 1993.

Tardive dyskinesia (TD) is a syndrome of extrapyramidal side effects. Symptoms of tardive dyskinesia are similar to those of dyskinesia except that they occur later in drug therapy. This late appearing side effect is characterized by abnormal, involuntary movements of the mouth, face, limbs, and trunk. Ten percent of the patients treated with antipsychotics develop TD (Julien, 1992). Among the chronically mentally ill, 26 percent of inpatients experience TD. Onset of TD is thought to be related to the patient's age and the drug's dose. Also, women are more likely than men to develop TD. Because TD is a potentially irreversible condition and its prevalence is increasing, antipsychotics should only be administered in appropriate situations. Additionally, because TD is dose-related, discovering a *minimum* effective dose is important (Jeste & Wyatt, 1982).

A very serious complication that can occur when using antipsychotic agents is **neuroleptic malignant syndrome** (NMS). NMS is like a severe form of Parkinson's, where the patient is catatonic (unable to move). Unstable blood pressure and heart rate, hyperthermia, mutism, and stupor are also part of this syndrome. Because NMS is sometimes fatal, intensive care is recommended. NMS is more likely to occur if the patient is also medically sick or has been taking many different antipsychotics, a situation referred to as **polypharmacy** (Caroff & Mann, 1988). After onset of NMS, the antipsychotic drug regime is immediately discontinued. Following a single occurrence and recovery from NMS, there is an 80 percent chance of NMS reoccurring with the reintroduction of antipsychotics (Olin et al., 1993).

DRUG INTERACTIONS AND TOXICITY

The fact that antipsychotics generally have a large therapeutic window makes them relatively safe drugs. Undesirable side effects of antipsychotic agents renders these drugs nonreinforcing. Therefore, this class of drugs in not likely to be abused (Baldessarini, 1993).

Because antipsychotics are highly protein bound, and remain in the bloodstream for a long time, the chance of interaction with other drugs is considerable (Olin et al., 1993). When selecting an antipsychotic agent, these factors should be considered:

- Side-effect profile
- History of previous response
- Dosage forms
- Need for sedation
- Other medication patient takes
- Presence of physical disease
- Patient compliance
- Patient's sex and body weight
- Stage and severity of the illness

Psychiatrists generally go through a "trial and error" ritual in prescribing antipsychotic agents.

CLASSIFICATION OF ANTIPSYCHOTIC DRUGS

PHENOTHIAZINES

All drugs in this category share the same basic chemical structure. Of all the antipsychotics, the **phenothiazines** are the oldest and the most prescribed (Ponterotto, 1985). Select phenothiazines are used as antiemetics (antivomiting) and have other labeled uses; many have unlabeled uses. Some agents are marketed under more than one trade name. Phenothiazines act at dopamine-1 and dopamine-2 receptors. The onset of therapeutic action is delayed, usually requiring four to six weeks for maximum neuroleptic effect (Olin et al., 1993). Here are some of the more popular phenothiazines:

Trade Name	Generic Name
Compazine	Prochlorperazine
Mellaril	Thioridazine
Permitil	Fluphenazine
Prolixin	Fluphenazine
Serentil	Mezoridazine
Sparine	Promazine
Stelazine	Trifluoperazine
Thorazine	Chlorpromazine
Tindal	Acetophenazine maleate
Trilafon	Perphenazine
Vesprin	Triflupromazine [Olin et al., 1993]

THIOXANTHENES

The chemical structure and effects of thioxanthenes are very similar to those of phenothiazines. They are very potent and effective agents (Baldessarini, 1993). The most common thioxanthenes include:

Trade Name	Generic Name
Navane	Thiothixene
Taractan	Chlorprothixene

OTHER ANTIPSYCHOTIC DRUGS

A number of other antipsychotic drugs worth mentioning here, including the following:

Trade Name	Generic Name
Clozaril	Clozapine
Haldol	Haloperidol
Loxitane	Loxapine
Moban	Molindone

Clozaril (clozapine) is chemically similar to loxapine but is considered to be an atypical antipsychotic agent. Clozaril acts on dopamine-1 receptors and also blocks serotonin. An advantage of Clozaril is that it is free of extrapyramidal side effects (EPS) and TD. Side effects are mainly anticholinergic. Because of a serious, potentially fatal adverse effect (agranulocytosis), Clozaril is not the drug of first choice in treating schizophrenia and must be prescribed with caution. Patients taking Clozaril must have weekly blood tests to detect the possible onset of agranulocytosis (Brenner et al., 1990; Olin et al., 1993). By itself, Clozaril is an extremely expensive drug, costing $4,160 annually. With the cost of the physician monitoring added, the cost can soar another $1,300 a year (Wallis & Willwerth, 1992).

Haldol (haloperidol) is the most potent of all the neuroleptics. It acts predominantly at dopamine-2 receptors. Haldol's adverse effects are primarily extrapyramidal side effects. However, of all the antipsychotics, its EPS are the greatest. Other labeled uses of Haldol include: (1) Tourette's disorder; (2) severe behavioral problems in children, such as combative explosive behavior that is unexplained by provocation; and (3) short-term use for hyperactive children. Anecdotal and unconfirmed evidence has surfaced that Asians may be more sensitive to this drug or are at higher risk for serious side effects or toxic reactions.

Loxitane (loxapine) is similar to the phenothiazines (Olin et al., 1993). Moban (molindone) produces less sedation than the other drugs in this category.

ANTI-PARKINSON AGENTS

Anti-Parkinson agents are often prescribed to counteract the induced extrapyramidal, Parkinson's-like effects of the phenothiazines and Haldol. Among the drugs in this category are:

Trade Name	Generic Name
Akineton	Biperiden
Artane	Trihexyphenidyl
Benadryl	Diphenhydramine
Cogentin	Benztropine
Kemadrin	Procyclidine
Parsidol	Ethopropazine
Symmetrel	Amantadine [Olin et al., 1993]

DRUGS THAT CAN PRODUCE PSYCHOTIC SYMPTOMS

Psychotic behavior is generally thought to result from a **functional disorder,** as in schizophrenia or depression. **Functional psychoses** are abnormal behaviors that cannot be attributed to any single known cause, whereas **organic psychoses** can result from a recognized insult to the brain, such as high fever or drug use (Price & Lynn, 1986). Almost every known drug has the potential to produce side effects that are manifested as psychotic behavior. Unfortunately, this abnormal behavior is often misdiagnosed as a functional disorder. The difficulty in making an accurate diagnosis relates to the increase in both illicit drug use and self-medication. Not only is the increase in illicit drug consumption a problem, but the underreporting in usage of both over-the-counter medication and prescription drugs adds to the confusion (Taylor, 1990). Additionally, separating a drug's side effects from the symptoms of the illness for which the therapeutic agent is administered can be challenging. In this section, therapeutic agents, which are common or are known for the severity of their side effects, will be discussed.

PSYCHOTOXIC DRUGS

Psychotoxic drugs alter the functioning of the central nervous system (CNS). Baldessarini (1985) divides psychotoxic drugs into three subcategories:

1. Therapeutic agents that have legitimate uses but also possess a significant potential for abuse. Drugs in this category include sedatives, stimulants, and opioid analgesics.
2. Drugs that have no established medical use but are popular in today's society. Examples in this group are caffeine, alcohol, tobacco, marijuana, and hallucinogens.
3. Drugs that are valued for their medicinal benefits but whose use brings about psychiatric side effects. Cardiac glycosides, antihypertensives, sedatives, stimulants, and steroids are members of this category.

We will not discuss drugs such as caffeine, tobacco, or others in the second grouping that lack any medically recognized benefits. Therapeutic agents with the potential for psychiatric adverse effects will be the focus. However, Baldessarini's (1985) third category can be expanded. Apparently, to be included in this grouping a drug must *directly affect* the CNS to produce psychotic behavior. We would be remiss if we omitted other drugs that *indirectly alter* normal CNS functioning such as agents that modify blood sugar levels or drugs that reduce cerebral blood flow. Therefore, we have also included drugs that indirectly alter CNS functioning.

SIDE EFFECTS. Drug therapy should not be initiated unless the anticipated benefits outweigh the drug's potential hazards. Although the drug industry and the health community have collaborated and made strides in increasing the reporting of adverse reactions, it is impossible to determine the exact probability or frequency of occurrence of a side effect. A higher incidence of adverse reactions has been reported in these specific populations: females, geriatrics, and patients with kidney problems (Tatro, Ow-Wing, & Huie, 1986).

Side effects generally result from the agent's nonselective receptor binding capacity. A drug circulating in the body will bind with any receptor that the drug's chemical structure will allow. Most therapeutic agents exert effects at other receptors in addition to the targeted receptor site. The majority of adverse effects are dose-related, meaning as the dose increases the number of side effects will also increase. Conversely, a decrease in dose usually decreases the magnitude of unwanted effects.

An **idiosyncratic reaction** is a type of side effect that occurs in only a very small percentage of the population. The exact mechanism of action for idiosyncratic reactions is not understood; however, it is suspected to be genetically related (Tatro et al., 1986).

PREDISPOSING FACTORS. Not all individuals who ingest a particular drug will exhibit psychiatric symptoms. This suggests that certain factors predispose development of a substance-induced psychotic disorder. Research has shown that genetic factors coupled with the stress of drug use can trigger a functional disorder. Suspected predisposing factors in drug-induced psychotic disorders are

- genetics, a family history of psychiatric disorders;
- personal history of functional disorder;
- physical illness, especially an illness that affects brain tissue (Gilderman, 1979); and
- individuals with a history of substance abuse (Taylor, 1990).

MECHANISMS OF DRUG-INDUCED PSYCHOSES. Exact drug mechanisms responsible for inducing psychotic behavior are not known. Researchers have advanced various theories. A popular hypothesis states that raised CNS dopamine (DA) levels cause psychotic behavior (for example, flight from reality, hallucinations, delusions, break between thought and action). Support for the dopamine hypothesis relates to a treatment for Parkinson's disease in which exogenous DA, L-Dopa, is administered. However, one unwanted side effect that sometimes occurs with administration of a dopamine drug is schizophrenic-like behavior. Despite the evidence of dopamine's involvement in psychotic behavior, the dopamine theory is regarded as an oversimplification because very high levels of other neurotransmitters (norepinephrine, for example) can also cause psychotic behavior. However, although other neurotransmitters and processes are also important in the development of psychosis, rises in dopamine clearly account for many of the psychotic symptoms.

DRUGS WITH ANTICHOLINERGIC PROPERTIES THAT CAN PRODUCE PSYCHOSIS

Drugs that block the effects of the neurotransmitter acetylcholine (ACh) in the body are described as having **anticholinergic properties.** Anticholinergic effects of drugs can occur in very small doses, especially in children and the elderly. If a patient is experiencing some of the CNS adverse effects from drug therapy along with physical side effects, it is likely that the aberrant behavior is drug-induced.

NON-CNS SIDE EFFECTS. Non-CNS side effects include decreased sweating, decreased salivation, dry mucous membranes, dilated pupils, facial flushing, tachycardia (increased heart rate), increased blood pressure, decreased bowel activity, and urinary hesitancy or retention (Brown, 1993).

CNS SIDE EFFECTS. CNS side effects include amnesia, delirium, disorientation, agitation, anxiety, paranoia, restlessness, mania, insomnia, drowsiness, and hallucinations (Brown, 1993). Box 4-2 contains further information on the various types of drugs that may have anticholinergic effects.

ANTI-PARKINSON AGENTS

Parkinson's disease is thought to result from an imbalance between two CNS neurotransmitters, ACh and DA. In this disease, dopaminergic neurons in the brain's substantia nigra are affected, causing a deficit of DA. Because DA and ACh are in opponent process, ACh gets the upper hand. Both exogenous DA and anticholinergics, which hold down ACh, are often prescribed for Parkinson's. An unwanted side effect that sometimes occurs with dopamine drugs is schizophrenic-like behavior.

NON-CNS SIDE EFFECTS. Non-CNS side effects include anorexia, nausea, vomiting, and dry mouth.

Box 4-2 Drugs with Anticholinergic Actions

Anti-Parkinson agents have anticholinergic actions. Here are some of the more useful drugs in this category:

Trade Name	Generic Name
Akineton	Biperiden
Artane	Trihexyphenidyl
Cogentin	Benzotropine
Kemadrin	Procyclidine
Parsidol	Ethopropazine

Antispasmodic drugs are used to treat gastrointestinal problems, including spastic colon, irritable bowel, mucous colitis, and others. This category of drugs includes:

Trade Name	Generic Name
Bentyl	Dicyclomine
Donnatal	Atropine, scopolamine, hyoscyamine
Levsin	L-hyoscyamine [Olin et al., 1993]

Antipsychotic agents listed previously in Chapter 4 also have anticholinergic actions.

Antihistamines do not all produce the same amount of anticholinergic activity. However, psychotic symptoms are usually only noted with large doses or overdoses.

Tricyclic antidepressants also have anticholinergic actions. For specific drug references, see Chapter 2.

CNS SIDE EFFECTS.   CNS side effects include depression with or without suicidal tendencies, hallucinations, delusions, agitation, anxiety, nightmares, euphoria, and dementia.

Useful drugs in this category include:

Trade Name	Generic Name
Larodopa	Levodopa
Parlodel	Bromocriptine
Sinemet	Carbidopa and levodopa
Symmetrel	Amantadine (also used to treat the influenza A virus) [Olin et al., 1993]

STIMULANTS

Stimulants are prescribed by doctors for obesity, attention-deficit disorder, and narcolepsy.

NON-CNS SIDE EFFECTS.   Non-CNS side effects include dilated pupils, increased heart rate and respiration, blood pressure changes, increased or decreased salivation, tremor, insomnia, and sweating (Maxmen, 1991).

CNS SIDE EFFECTS.   CNS side effects include anxiety, agitation, irritability, aggression, confusion, paranoid hallucinations, panic states, and suicidal or homicidal tendencies (Hoffman & Lefkowitz, 1993). The psychotic episodes that can occur with stimulants clinically resembles paranoid schizophrenia behavior.

Amphetamine stimulants include the following:

Trade Name	Generic Name
Dexedrine	Dextroamphetamine
Desoxyn	Methamphetamine

Nonamphetamine anorexiant agents are appetite suppressors and include the following:

Trade Name	Generic Name
Fastin	Phentermine
Ionamin	Phentermine
Preludin	Phenmetrazine [Olin et al., 1993]

OPIOID ANALGESICS

Opioid analgesics or narcotics are controlled substances that physicians prescribe for moderate to severe pain. Morphine is the prototype of the opioid analgesic class of drugs. Effects of narcotic analgesics can be potentiated by the intake of other CNS depressants, including alcohol, BZDs (valium-like drugs), or other narcotics.

NON-CNS SIDE EFFECTS.   Non-CNS side effects include nausea, vomiting, and sweating (all of which are most prominent in ambulatory patients who are not experiencing severe pain), constipation, abdominal cramps, urinary hesitancy or retention, and decreased blood pressure.

CNS SIDE EFFECTS. CNS side effects include dizziness, sedation, insomnia, anxiety, fear, agitation, euphoria, dysphoria, disorientation, and hallucinations (Olin et al., 1993). Specific opioid analgesics are discussed in Chapter 5.

DIGITALIS GLYCOSIDES

Digitalis glycosides are derived from plants and are used to treat heart problems.

NON-CNS SIDE EFFECTS. Non-CNS side effects include anorexia, nausea, vomiting, diarrhea, and cardiac arrhythmias.

CNS SIDE EFFECTS. CNS side effects include disorientation, confusion, delirium, fatigue, headaches, aphasia, distraction, bizarre thoughts, paranoid delusions, and hallucinations. The best-known drug in this category is Digoxin (lanoxin) and there are very few others (Olin et al., 1993).

CORTICOSTEROIDS

Corticosteroids are used systemically to treat endocrine disorders, rheumatic disorders, collagen diseases, dermatologic diseases, gastrointestinal disorders, nervous system disorders (multiple sclerosis), some cancers, and allergic states (Olin et al., 1993).

NON-CNS SIDE EFFECTS. Non-CNS side effects include fluid retention, weight gain, increased appetite, impaired wound healing, menstrual irregularities, and **hirsutism** (coarsening of body hair).

CNS SIDE EFFECTS. CNS side effects include **steroid psychosis,** which is characterized by paranoid ideations, hallucinations, and a clouded sensorium. Other symptoms noted with steroid use are mood swings (euphoria or depression), personality changes, and insomnia. Onset of symptoms usually occurs within 15 to 30 days.

The occurrence of steroid psychosis does not correlate well with a history of psychiatric disorders. The incidence of this disorder is dose-related. One study revealed that of the 718 patients treated with prednisone at a daily dose of 40 mg or less, 1.3 percent experienced steroid psychosis. Yet at a daily dose of prednisone of 80 mg or more, 4.6 percent of the patients were afflicted with this psychosis. Symptoms remit with dose reductions. Antipsychotic medications can be used to control these symptoms when steroid therapy cannot be discontinued or the dose cannot be greatly reduced.

Only the systemic steroids or drugs that can be administered orally are listed here:

Trade Name   *Generic Name*
Aristocort   Triamcinolone
Delta-Cortef   Prednisolone
Deltasone   Prednisone
Medrol   Methylprednisolone
Orasone   Prednisone [Olin et al., 1993]

ANABOLIC STEROIDS

Anabolic steroids are closely related to the male hormone androgen. These drugs are very popular among competing athletes and body builders because they increase aggressiveness and muscle mass, decrease muscle recovery time after a weight lifting exercise, and decrease healing time after muscle injury. Despite their widespread use, anabolic steroids have only a few approved therapeutic uses. The FDA has approved their use in certain types of anemia, some forms of breast cancer, and for hereditary angioedema (Olin et al., 1993).

NON-CNS SIDE EFFECTS. Non-CNS side effects include acne, nausea, vomiting, yellowing of eyes and skin. In females, additional side effects include menstrual irregularities, deepening and hoarseness of the voice, male pattern baldness, and hirsutism. In males, additional side effects include early balding and development of enlarged breasts (Olin et al., 1993).

CNS SIDE EFFECTS. CNS side effects include depression, insomnia, excitation (Olin et al., 1993), mania, and psychosis (Abramowicz, 1990).

CNS DEPRESSANTS

Psychotic behavior can occur during treatment with CNS depressants or during withdrawal from CNS depressants. However, problems are more likely to arise when the sedative-hypnotic or depressant drug is discontinued. The two main categories of CNS depressants are barbiturates and benzodiazepines. Both classes of drugs have been prescribed for sleep problems and anxiety states. For specific drugs in both classes, refer to the listings in Chapter 3.

NON-CNS SIDE EFFECTS. Non-CNS side effects include delirium tremens–like syndrome that appears upon withdrawal.

CNS SIDE EFFECTS. CNS side effects include rage, hostility, paranoia, hallucinations, depression, insomnia, and nightmares (Abramowicz, 1990).

BETA-ADRENERGIC BLOCKING AGENTS

Beta-adrenergic blocking agents (beta-blockers) are a group of structurally related compounds used to treat hypertension, migraines, and a variety of heart problems (Olin et al., 1993). Many problems can occur with the usual dose (Abramowicz, 1990).

NON-CNS SIDE EFFECTS. Non-CNS side effects include dry mouth, nausea, vomiting, headaches, and lethargy.

CNS SIDE EFFECTS. CNS side effects include depression, confusion, nightmares, insomnia, dizziness, anxiety, hallucinations, and paranoia.

Beta blockers include the drugs listed here:

Trade Name	Generic Name
Blocadren	Timolol
Brevibloc	Esmolol
Cartrol	Carteolol
Corgard	Nadolol
Inderal	Propranolol
Kerlone	Betaxolol
Levatol	Penbutolol
Lopressor	Metoprolol
Normodyne	Labetalol
Tenormin	Atenolol
Sectral	Acebutolol
Visken	Pindolol [Olin et al., 1993]

DRUG-INDUCED DEPRESSION

Short-term symptoms of a drug-induced depression are indistinguishable from those of a primary or endogenous depression. However, some chronic physical illnesses or genetic factors can predispose an individual to a drug-induced depression. Even though depression is frequently noted in individuals who take CNS depressants, it should not be assumed that the CNS depressant is the primary cause of the depression (Swonger & Matejski, 1991).

DRUGS THAT CAN PRODUCE DEPRESSION

HYPERTENSIVES. An antihypertensive agent has the ability to prevent or control high blood pressure. Some common drugs in this category include:

Trade Name	Generic Name
Aldomet	Methyldopa
Catapres	Clonidine
Inderal	Propanolol
Ismelin	Guanethidine
Lopressor	Metoprolol
Minipress	Prazosin
Serpasil	Reserpine (Fuller & Underwood, 1989)

Reserpine is an older antihypertensive agent and is contraindicated in patients with a history of affective disorders. Depression occurs in a significant percentage of people who use reserpine (7–20 percent). Reserpine-induced depression can persist for several months after the drug is discontinued, and the depression may be severe enough to end in suicide (Olin et al., 1993).

ORAL CONTRACEPTIVES. The incidence of depression in females taking birth control pills ranges between 5 and 30 percent. A history of depression appears to be a predisposing factor. Excessive progestin is thought to cause depression. Discontinuation of the oral contraceptives is the usual treatment for this type of depression (Olin et al., 1993).

WITHDRAWAL FROM STIMULANTS. It is not uncommon for individuals who have used appetite suppressants chronically to experience depression when the stimulant drug is discontinued. Refer to the drugs listed under stimulants in the previous section for names of drugs in this group.

MISCELLANEOUS. Indocin (Indomethacin) is a nonsteroidal anti-inflammatory agent used in the treatment of certain types of arthritis, bursitis, and gout. Indocin is not only noted for causing depression but may also aggravate other psychiatric disturbances (Olin et al., 1993).

DRUG-INDUCED ORGANIC BRAIN SYNDROME

Approximately 20 percent of the admissions in psychiatric hospitals are patients diagnosed with **organic brain syndrome (OBS).** OBS is used to describe an assortment of conditions characterized by impaired brain functioning without indicating the etiology of the impairment (Swonger & Matejski, 1991). CNS impairment in OBS interferes with one or more of the following brain processes: memory (recent or remote), orientation, consciousness, intellect, insight, judgment, thought content (hallucinations or illusions), or mood (Thomas, 1985).

Many different types of OBS have been identified. OBS can be reversible (acute) or irreversible (chronic). Dementia and delirium are two global forms of OBS. **Dementia** refers to the loss of intellectual ability that results in impairment in occupational and social functioning. About 20 percent of dementias are reversible, and this statistic needs to be communicated to patients' families. Alzheimer's disease is an example of an irreversible, degenerative dementia that is not drug-induced. Differing from dementia, **delirium** is a state of clouded consciousness, where an individual is unable to focus or sustain attention. Perceptual disturbances, hallucinations and illusions, sleep and affective disturbances, disorientation, and memory impairment are all components of delirium (APA, 1994). Other types of OBS with specific etiologies have been identified. One example is *amnesic syndrome* (Wernicke-Korsakoff), which results from vitamin B1 deficiency seen in alcoholism (Swonger & Matejski, 1991).

Numerous mechanisms are responsible for producing OBS symptoms. Such mechanisms can occur in certain drug therapies or in the interaction of a drug with a medical disorder. Components of a disease process, such as fever, infections, inflammatory conditions, brain lesions, or brain tumors, can also produce OBS symptoms. Some drugs can act directly on CNS tissue and alter its functioning. Indirect drug mechanisms that can produce OBS include:

- inadequate brain oxygen caused by decreased cerebral blood flow due to a reduction in cardiac output or blood pressure, and
- decreased brain glucose use resulting from low blood sugar (Taylor, 1990).

DRUGS THAT CAN CAUSE OBS

A variety of drugs can cause organic brain syndrome, among them are drugs that cause hypotension, diuretics, hypoglycemic agents, drugs with anticholinergic properties, and sedative-hypnotic drugs.

DRUGS THAT CAUSE HYPOTENSION. Many drugs and categories of drugs have hypotensive properties, the ability to reduce blood pressure. Significant reductions in blood pressure may lead to obvious confusion and disorientation. Geriatrics are especially vulnerable to the hypotensive effects of drugs. Classes of drugs with hypotensive properties include antihypertensives, antipsychotics, tricyclic antidepressants, monoamine oxidase inhibitor antidepressants, and narcotics (Swonger & Matejski, 1991).

DIURETICS. A **diuretic** is a drug that increases the amount of urine excreted by the kidney. Mental functioning can be impaired by overdiuresis (excessive fluid and electrolyte loss). The confusion, lethargy, dizziness, and anxiety caused by diuretics can be reversed by discontinuing the agents and correcting the fluid and electrolyte abnormalities (Swonger & Matejski, 1991). Individuals with eating disorders often abuse diuretics to achieve higher weight loss and need to be closely monitored.

HYPOGLYCEMIC AGENTS. **Hypoglycemic agents** are drugs that have the ability to lower the blood sugar level in the body. Reductions in blood sugar caused by dosage errors in insulin and oral hypoglycemics can be so drastic that bizarre behavior, slurred speech, irrational fear, delusions, hallucinations, and mental confusion may occur (Taylor, 1990).

DRUGS WITH ANTICHOLINERGIC PROPERTIES. Besides having the potential for inducing psychotic behavior, drugs with anticholinergic properties may also precipitate a state of delirium. This unwanted confusional state is more likely to occur in the geriatric population. Therefore, anticholinergic agents should be prescribed with caution to the elderly (Taylor, 1990).

SEDATIVE-HYPNOTIC DRUGS. Geriatric patients and individuals with preexisting organic problems are especially vulnerable to the sedative effects of hypnotics, tranquilizers (anxiolytics), antipsychotics, tricyclic antidepressants, and antihistamines. For this reason, conservative use is recommended in these susceptible populations (Swonger & Matejski, 1991).

5

PAIN AND THE ANALGESICS

The experience of pain involves both an awareness of an uncomfortable sensation and an emotional reaction to the hurting episode. Pain is more than a sensory experience; it is an emotional experience that can have lasting effects on the psyche. The emotional and sensory components of pain are mediated through different centers in the brain (Melzack, 1986). The cognitive representations of the hurting episodes, the anticipation of how the discomfort will affect the future, and the emotional background and immediate "surround" all have an impact on the experience of pain. It is for these reasons, and because clients taking pain medications are often seen in psychotherapy, that we have included pain medications.

Chronic back pain, the most expensive single pain complaint, is an excellent example of a usually acute injury that often leads to psychological referral for a chronically painful condition. Altmaier and Johnson (1992) provide the following summary:

- Eighty percent of adults will have significant low back pain, and about 30 percent of them will seek medical attention. Of this medical use group, 35 percent will be pain free in one month, 70 percent pain free in two months, 86 percent pain free in three months, and 96 percent pain free in one year.
- The approximately 3 percent who are disabled include 75,000 workers.
- The total expense for all back injuries in health care costs, disability payments, lost work, and lawsuits totaled $60 billion in 1977, and 25 percent of the injury cases accounted for around 87 percent of the total costs.

The overall expenditure of one dollar for counseling among this medical group saves approximately three dollars in future medical costs. Unfortunately, psychotherapy and rehabilitation counseling (by a trained rehabilitation counselor as opposed to a hospital worker with rehabilitation experience) is too often seen as a last resort rather than as an ordinary complement to physical rehabilitation.

UNDERSTANDING THE CHARACTERISTICS OF PAIN

Pain is considered useful in that it is an informative process responsible for alerting the body to a harmful condition. It is, therefore, an adaptive mechanism. In the disease model, treatment of pain focuses on removal of the underlying cause (Berntzen & Gotestam, 1987). However, intensive medical and surgical approaches often fail to uncover the etiology of pain. This is often the case with **chronic pain,** which lasts longer than three months and is often not directly associated with continuing tissue damage (Supernaw, 1991a). Chronic pain resulting from progressive malignancies, neuropathies, arthritic conditions, and other states have identifiable sources and are frequently treated more aggressively than chronic pain without a known etiology. Supernaw (1991a) purports that **acute pain** usually lasts less than 30 days and is deemed functional.

Chronic pain frequently originates as an acute episode, then evolves into a prolonged condition. Unfortunately, treatment attempts such as multiple surgeries (and the numerous narcotic prescriptions that accompany them) often exacerbate chronic pain states by adding further injury, scar tissue, and nerve damage to the original site. The majority of chronic pain conditions persist for years in contrast with the short-lived placebo effects of some medications. After numerous treatment attempts, chronic pain sufferers are suspected of not experiencing "real pain"—even though their pain is the product of physical insult—and psychotherapy is belatedly recommended.

Pain without specific etiology or background insult is frequently labeled *psychogenic* (Fordyce & Steger, 1979). Physicians sometimes confuse psychogenic pain and chronic pain, assuming that an injury that has "healed" should no longer cause pain unless that pain produces some secondary gain. Why pain continues to be produced in old injury sites is not completely clear. Pain specialists have found, however, that the nerves that send pain impulses are sensitized in such a way that they continue to send higher levels of impulses than are warranted by the healing injury.

Berntzen and Gotestam (1987) make a similar distinction between types of pain but employ different terms. *Respondent pain* follows tissue damage, whereas *operant pain* may or may not result from tissue damage. Another distinguishing factor is that the behavior involved in operant pain may be reinforced by either social attention or by reduction of tension, fear, or anxiety. Most pain includes both respondent and operant events. The psychological and emotional consequences of chronic pain are often experienced as suffering—feelings of hopelessness, despair, and anxiety—all of which reflect the subjective experience of pain (Fordyce & Steger, 1979).

Physical pain with a purely psychogenic origin is rare. Physical pain that continues after an acute injury episode is over is very common. Injury to the body through stress-related factors and their painful aftermath (ulcers, for example), is also quite common. Psychological problems cause physical problems that cause pain and that exacerbate pain from injuries. The mind, however, rarely creates pain out of whole cloth, without an underlying physical referent.

In the same way that doctors and other health care workers often underestimate their patients' unwillingness to adopt better health care practices (for example, quitting smoking), they often overestimate the ability of patients to resolve chronic pain conditions without psychological help and without the onus that they, themselves, by virtue of some psychological dysfunction, are causing the pain to continue long after it should have stopped. Blaming the victim magnifies the problems patients have and makes it more difficult to treat the psychological component of their pain reaction.

It should be emphasized that most patients with chronic pain who are successfully treated psychologically do not significantly reduce their pain levels even though they come to terms with their physical problem and are in good mental health. It is likely that successful psychological treatment accounts for no more than 20 percent of the variance in the experience of pain; the other 80 percent is the result of dimensions of the pain experience that we simply do not understand at this point in our medical knowledge.

Diagnosis of the etiology and ramifications of present pain is of crucial importance in later treatment. Patients who have been told or led to believe that their pain is all in their head make very difficult counseling clients, not only because this view is false in a vast majority of cases but also because it undermines trust in the therapeutic relationship by blaming the patient.

A MULTIDISCIPLINARY APPROACH TO TREATMENT

In an effort to obtain a cure, chronic pain patients tend to overutilize the medical system (Deardoff, Rubin, & Scott, 1991). Berntzen and Gotestam (1987) contend that pain behavior is positively reinforced by pain medications. Whether or not the pain behavior is reinforced, it is clear that chronic, low-level pain does not respond well to management with morphine or its synthetic derivatives and tolerance to and dependence on them grow very rapidly. Clearly, over time drug therapy for chronic, non–life-threatening pain can lead to increased use and to addiction.

Chronic pain is maintained by multiple factors, therefore multidisciplinary rather than unidimensional treatment is recommended. Prototypical multidisciplinary pain programs involve active physical therapy, stress and anxiety management, body mechanics and posture training, relaxation and self-regulating procedures, biofeedback, pain medication reduction, and individual or group counseling (Deardoff et al., 1991). Deardoff et al. (1991) conducted a study comparing the effects of a comprehensive multidisciplinary treatment program for a group of chronic pain patients with a group of chronic pain sufferers who received no treatment. Results showed that the multidisciplinary approach was more effective in producing increased physical functioning, decreased drug use, and an increase in the "return to work" rate. The no treatment group did not experience similar improvements. However, there were no differences between the two groups in their subjective experiences of pain. Therefore, the primary goal of multidisciplinary pain programs is to increase functioning and return to normalcy (reduction of suffering). Pain reduction (reduction of pain perception) is an important but secondary goal. Clearly, pain perception does not need to lead to subjective suffering!

Tension headaches cause chronic pain for many individuals. Supernaw (1991b) recommends behavior modification, eliminating tension-causing ingredients such as caffeine from the diet, and investigating the possible precipitating roles anxiety and depression may play in the occurrence of tension headaches. Other underlying psychiatric processes may also be at work and should be investigated if behavioral techniques do not provide incremental relief.

STRATEGIES FOR DELIVERY OF ANALGESICS

Counselors may work with clients who are in severe or progressive pain situations. In these situations, new strategies for delivery of analgesics and dosing schedules are useful, and we will include them in this discussion.

Physicians frequently prescribe pain medications on a PRN basis. **PRN** means *pro re nata* or that medications are given on demand or as needed (Berntzen & Gotestam, 1987). Yet PRN analgesic administration is problematic. With chronic pain sufferers as subjects, Berntzen and Gotestam (1987) conducted a study comparing the effects of PRN (pain-contingent) dosing with fixed interval (time contingent) dosing. Results indicate that a fixed interval schedule is more effective in controlling pain and improving mood. Further, fixed interval dosing regimens are believed to have a lower potential for drug dependence.

Supernaw (1991a) indicates that in severe pain, PRN dosing allows the pain to return before redosing is initiated and that more drug therefore may be used with PRN dosing regimens. Furthermore, employing a regular or fixed administration schedule of pain medication prevents the occurrence of pain memory. Once the pain reappears, the patient begins to anticipate pain distress, which can increase the emotional reaction, thus elevating the experience of pain.

Patient-controlled analgesia (PCA) is a well-accepted pain management technique. As the name implies, patients control the frequency of the analgesic administration. Usually used in hospital settings, PCA devices consist of a pump that is activated by the patient to initiate infusion of small doses of narcotics into an intravenous catheter. The safety of PCA from overdose is ensured by a built-in mechanism or system of constraints. Drug concentration levels in the blood fluctuate minimally with PCA administration devices, therefore the peak sedative effects do not occur as often (Bedder, Soifer, & Mulhall, 1991). An added psychological benefit with PCA devices is that the patient is empowered by having the ability to help combat an adverse experience.

In treating a variety of medical conditions such as hypertension, physicians routinely begin with a low dosage and then increase the dose until the desired effect is achieved. Yet, in severe acute pain situations, an aggressive dosing philosophy called *descending the ladder* is recommended. With this dosing method, the starting dose is slightly tapered downward until the patient's pain threshold is discovered. The advantage to this type of dosing philosophy is that the patient's pain is relieved rapidly rather than gradually. The speedy removal of discomfort helps lower the patient's anxiety or emotional reaction, thereby helping to alleviate the experience of pain (Supernaw, 1991a). When a patient's dose of narcotics must be increased to maintain pain relief, as sometimes occurs with progressive malignancies, the sedative side effects of the narcotic may be combatted with amphetamine stimulants or methylphenidate (Ritalin).

HEADACHE PAIN

Of all the recurrent medical conditions, headaches are the most common and the most annoying. A variety of chronic or recurrent headache types are described in the literature. Health care workers note that the *tension headache* (also referred to as stress, muscle contraction, or ordinary headache) produces the most frequent complaints and plagues 10 to 20 percent of the population. Without any warning signs, tension headaches begin with gradual dull and nagging pain affecting both sides of the head (Supernaw, 1991b).

Although not as common as the tension type, *migraine headaches* receive the most attention. A migraine is a vascular headache that produces intense pain lasting 4 to 12 hours; it is often preceded by a prodromal sign. It is caused by dilation of cranial vessels and may put pressure on the optic nerve. Most of the time, migraine pain occurs on only one side of the head. Patients may also experience nausea, vomiting, and diarrhea. Hypersensitivity to lights or sound can also occur with migraines. Additionally, physical exertion has been shown to aggravate a migraine headache. A genetic component may be involved, for migraines are known to run in families (Supernaw, 1991b).

Some of the agents used in the treatment and prevention of migraine headaches have not been mentioned yet. An ergot alkaloid drug (ergotamine) causes constriction of cranial blood vessels and is valuable in aborting and preventing migraines. Ergot alkaloids are toxic drugs, therefore they should only be taken as prescribed by a physician. A related drug, methysergide, is used only as a prophylactic for migraine or vascular headaches. Two other agents, timolol and propanolol, are also helpful in preventing migraines. These two drugs are members of a group of drugs called beta-blockers, which are better known for their cardiovascular effects. Finally, drugs that raise levels of 5-HT successfully treat many migraine sufferers. Samatriptan (Imitrex), as well as the heterocyclic AMs, are becoming more widely used.

PAIN PATHWAYS

To understand how analgesics work, you must be acquainted with the body's pain pathways. Pain receptors in the skin are referred to as **nociceptors**. When nociceptors are stimulated with noxious stimuli, messages are sent to the spinal cord where the neurotransmitter substance P is released. Substance P sends the pain messages to brain centers by way of two neural pain pathways. These two ascending pain pathways are responsible for the sensory component during a painful experience, whereas the pain's emotional aspect is mediated by the limbic system (Carlson, 1991; Julien, 1992).

The body also has built-in mechanisms to combat the sensation of pain. Two descending inhibitory pain (or analgesic) pathways have been identified. One analgesic pathway originates in the locus caeruleus (located in the medulla of the brain). Activation of this pathway causes the release of the neurotransmitter NE in the spinal cord. NE acts to inhibit the release of substance P, thereby producing an analgesic effect. The brain's second natural analgesic pathway begins in the midbrain and medulla, ultimately affecting delivery of serotonin in the spinal cord. In the spinal cord, serotonin triggers the release of endogenous opioids, which in turn inhibit liberation of substance P. Considering the mechanisms involved in the two descending inhibitory pain pathways, drugs that increase the body's serotonin or potentiate NE (antidepressants, for example) have analgesic effects (Julien, 1992).

CHRONIC PAIN IN THE ELDERLY

Chronic pain is common in the elderly because of the high prevalence of arthritis, cancer, and vascular disease in this population, yet analgesic prescription and drug use declines with advancing age. The reasons for this reduction are not clear. Nevertheless, because of specific factors associated with aging such as reduced liver and kidney functioning, reduced body mass, and gastric atrophy, the elderly have an increased risk for analgesic toxicity.

TREATMENT WITH NARCOTICS

A notable feature of an analgesic state is that it can occur without a loss of consciousness (Jaffe & Martin, 1985). Analgesic agents, drugs that reduce sensitivity to pain, can be globally categorized into narcotics or non-narcotics. In severe acute or chronic pain with a known etiology, narcotics are frequently prescribed.

Other terms used to refer to narcotic analgesics are **opioids** or **opiates**. Opioids are naturally occurring (endogenous or exogenous) or synthetic drugs that mimic the effects of morphine. Morphine or other similar drugs are extracted from the opium poppy. Dating back to ancient cultures, opium has been used for a variety of different reasons, including both medicinal and recreational purposes. Endogenous opioids, those produced in the body and brain to aid in pain relief, are grouped into three distinct categories: enkephalins, endorphins, and dynorphins. Like their endogenous counterparts, morphine and morphine-like drugs collectively have a wide range of (mostly) inhibitory effects.

The targeted therapeutic or primary effect of narcotics is analgesia. However, these drugs have been associated with a variety of secondary pharmacological effects or side effects. The most frequently noted side effects are as follows:

System	Effects
CNS	Euphoria, drowsiness, apathy, mental confusion
Gastrointestinal	Constipation, nausea, vomiting
Cardiovascular	Hypotension (decrease in blood pressure) that may produce lightheadedness and fainting
Other	Urinary retention

The most hazardous side effect is respiratory depression, which is dose-dependent, can be potentiated by other CNS depressants, and can be fatal (Olin et al., 1993).

MECHANISMS OF ACTION

Chemical structures of morphine or synthetic narcotic agents closely resemble the chemical structures of the endogenous opioids, internal neuromodulators whose main duty is alleviation of physical and mental pain. This resemblance accounts for the narcotic drugs' stimulation of opioid receptors and the concomitant production of an analgesic state. A variety of opioid analgesics are known to exist, and not every opioid drug will produce all of these effects. Opioid analgesics differ in their molecular shape and their ability to stimulate specific opioid receptors (Jaffe & Martin, 1993).

Five major categories of opioid receptors have been identified; they are *mu, kappa, sigma, delta*, and *epsilon*. Table 5-1 lists the opioid receptors along with the usual effects of their stimulation.

Opioid drugs exert their effects by activating CNS opioid receptors located in the spinal cord, the brain stem, and the limbic system. The analgesic effect of opioids involve not only an alteration in sensation of pain but changes in affective responses to the pain. The action of several different systems of neurotransmitters (for example,

Table 5-1   Opioid Receptors and Their Effects

Receptor	Location	Effects
Mu	Supraspinal (thalamus, brain stem areas including locus caeruleus)	Analgesia, euphoria, respiratory depression, physical depression
Kappa	Spinal cord	Analgesia, sedation, miosis (pinpoint pupils)
Sigma	Limbic system	Dysphoria, psychotomimetic effects (such as hallucination)
Delta	Limbic system	Possible mood effect

Sources: Carlson, 1991; Julien, 1992; Olin et al., 1993.

norepinephrine and serotonin effects on substance-P) are components of the analgesic effects of narcotics (Jaffe & Martin, 1993).

CLASSIFICATION OF NARCOTIC ANALGESICS

Opioid drugs are classified as agonists, antagonists (or pure antagonists), or mixed agonist–antagonists.

NARCOTIC AGONISTS

If a drug stimulates an opioid receptor, producing morphine-like actions, the drug is referred to as an *agonist*. Narcotic agonists activate mu receptors, and to a lesser extent activate the kappa and sigma opioid receptors (Julien, 1992). Some narcotic agonists are naturally occurring compounds (for example, morphine and codeine); others are synthetic or semisynthetic drugs. Table 5-2 lists the more popular narcotic agonists.

In the 1800s, *Brompton's Mixture* was used as a pain cocktail for people suffering from progressive pain such as that associated with cancer. It was an amalgamation of morphine, cocaine, chloroform, and alcohol. Today's pain cocktail usually contains only morphine and is often referred to as a *Hospice Mixture* (Supernaw, 1991a). Sometimes other ingredients, such as aspirin, Tylenol, tricyclic antidepressants, antihistamines, or stimulants may be included (Olin et al., 1993).

To decrease the dose of narcotic agents or to increase the effectiveness of less potent analgesics, it is common for Tylenol (acetaminophen) or aspirin to be combined with a narcotic. It is important to be aware of narcotic analgesic

Table 5-2 Narcotic Agonists

Trade Name	Generic Name	Other Information
Codeine	Codeine	Also used as a cough suppressant
Darvon	Propoxyphene	In excessive doses has been associated with drug-related deaths
Demerol	Meperidine	
Dilaudid	Hydromorphone	
Dolophine	Methadone	Also used in detoxification programs
Duragesic	Fentanyl	Transdermal system skin patch worn for 72 hours
Levo-Dromoran	Levorphanol	
MS Contin	Morphine	A controlled release tablet
Opium Tincture	Paregoric	Mostly used as an antidiarrhea drug
Roxanol	Morphine	
Roxicodone	Oxycodone	

Note: Drugs available only in injectable or suppository form are not listed.

Source: Olin et al., 1993.

combinations because of their potential for abuse and depressive effects. Table 5-3 lists narcotic analgesic combinations that are frequently prescribed.

NARCOTIC ANTAGONISTS

Narcotic antagonist drugs can bind with opioid receptors but do not produce analgesic activity. These agents block the effects of narcotic agonists and can precipitate withdrawal in narcotic drug-dependent individuals. Obviously, narcotic antagonists are not used as analgesics. Table 5-4 lists the two drugs in this grouping, along with their uses.

MIXED AGONIST–ANTAGONIST ANALGESICS

Mixed agonist–antagonist drugs can stimulate some opioid receptors while blocking others. Most of these agents have an affinity for activating sigma

Table 5-3   Frequently Prescribed Narcotic Analgesic Combinations

Trade Name	Components
Darvocet-N 50	propoxyphene 50mg/acetaminophen 325mg
Darvocet-N 100	propoxyphene 100mg/acetaminophen 650mg
Darvon-N w/ASA	propoxyphene 100mg/aspirin 325mg
Darvon Compound	propoxyphene 32mg/aspirin 389mg/caffeine 32.4mg
Darvon Compound 65	propoxyphene 65mg/aspirin 389mg/caffeine 32.4mg
Empirin/Cod #2	codeine 15mg/aspirin 325mg
Empirin/Cod #3	codeine 30mg/aspirin 325mg
Empirin/Cod #4	codeine 60mg/aspirin 325mg
Fiorinal/Cod #3	codeine 30mg/acetaminophen 325mg/caffeine 40mg/ butalbital 50mg
Lortab	hydrocodone 2.5mg
Lortab 5	hydrocodone 5mg/acetaminophen 500mg
Lortab 7	hydrocodone 7.5mg/acetaminophen 500mg
Mepergan Fortis	meperidine 50mg/promethazine 25mg
Percodan	oxycodone 5mg/aspirin 325mg
Percocet	oxycodone 5mg/acetaminophen 325mg
Phenaphen/Cod #2	codeine 15mg/acetaminophen 325mg
Phenaphen/Cod #3	codeine 30mg/acetaminophen 325mg
Phenaphen 650/Cod	codeine 30mg/acetaminophen 650mg
Phenaphen/Cod #4	codeine 60mg/acetaminophen 325mg
Synalgos-DC	dihydrocodeine 16mg/aspirin 356.4mg
Tylenol/Cod #1	codeine 7.5mg/acetaminophen 300mg
Tylenol/Cod #2	codeine 15mg/acetaminophen 300mg
Tylenol/Cod #3	codeine 30mg/ acetaminophen 300 mg
Tylenol/Cod #4	codeine 60mg/acetaminophen 300mg
Tylox	oxycodone 5mg/acetaminophen 500mg
Wygesic	propoxyphene 65mg/acetaminophen 650mg

Source: Olin et al., 1993.

Table 5-4 Narcotic Antagonists and Their Uses

Trade Name	Generic Name	Use
Narcan	Naloxane drug	Treat narcotic overdoses
Trexan	Naltrexone	Help maintain an opioid-free state in detoxified opioid-dependent individuals

Source: Olin et al., 1993.

receptors, which can result in dysphoric and hallucinogenic experiences (Julien, 1992). An advantage this group of narcotic analgesics has is that it has a lower potential for abuse (Olin et al., 1993). Also, Supernaw (1991a) purports that these agents produce less respiratory depression. However, they are not recommended in progressive pain situations because of their low therapeutic dose ceiling. The agonist–antagonist drugs are:

Trade Name	Generic Name
Stadol NS	Butorphanol
Talwin	Pentazocine

OTHER ANALGESICS

SALICYLATE ANALGESICS

Aspirin, the most famous salicylate analgesic, was introduced in 1899 (Insel, 1993). Besides being effective in treating mild to moderate pain, it is an effective agent in inflammatory processes, including tissue damage and arthritic-like conditions. Aspirin is also valued for its antipyretic (fever reducing) action. Because aspirin inhibits blood platelet aggregation, lengthening blood clotting time, it is useful in preventing myocardial infarctions (heart attack).

Aspirin's analgesic activity is attributed to its effect on inhibiting prostaglandin synthesis. Being highly bound to proteins in the blood, aspirin's potential for interactions with other drugs is considerable. Gastrointestinal (GI) problems such as nausea, anorexia, and GI bleeding are the most frequent side effects associated with aspirin use. For this reason, it is recommended that aspirin be taken with food (Olin et al., 1993). Aspirin has the advantage over narcotic analgesics of being a nonaddictive agent. The average dose of aspirin will vary with the condition for which it is prescribed or indicated; however a common adult dose is one to two tablets (325 mg each) every four hours as needed. The usual adult dose is provided as a basis for comparison with the approximate acute lethal dose for adults, which is 10,000 mg to 30,000 mg (approximate lethal dose for children is 4,000 mg). Ear problems, such as dizziness or tinnitus (ringing in ears), are early warning signs of aspirin toxicity (Olin et al., 1993).

ACETAMINOPHEN

Tylenol (acetaminophen) is a viable alternative for individuals who should not take aspirin. It is equipotent to aspirin's analgesic and antipyretic effects. However, acetaminophen is void of anti-inflammatory properties, so its scope of usefulness is less than that of aspirin.

Acetaminophen's mechanism of action for its analgesic effect is not completely clear, but acetaminophen, like aspirin, inhibits prostaglandin synthesis in the CNS. However, in the peripheral nervous system, its ability to inhibit prostaglandin synthesis is minimal (Olin et al., 1993). Because it is metabolized in the liver, acetaminophen should be used with caution in individuals with liver problems. High doses of acetaminophen (5,000 mg or more per day, approximately ten extra-strength tablets) for two to three weeks have resulted in extensive liver damage and even death (Supernaw, 1991a).

NONSTEROIDAL ANTI-INFLAMMATORY DRUGS (NSAIDs)

NSAIDs are widely used, and the selection of a specific agent is determined by the physician and the nature of the problem. Although not more effective than aspirin, NSAIDs are recommended when pain is nonresponsive to aspirin therapy (Supernaw, 1991a). Egbert (1991) claims that the analgesic activity of NSAIDs is similar to that of weak narcotic analgesics such as propoxyphene (Darvon). NSAIDs possess anti-inflammatory, antipyretic, and analgesic activity. The exact mode of action is not known, but their ability to inhibit prostaglandin synthesis is important. Similar to aspirin, the major drawback of NSAID usage is GI problems. Also, these drugs are highly protein bound, so the potential for drug interactions is significant. Drowsiness, dizziness, and blurred vision are included in NSAIDs' side effects. Therefore, when taking NSAIDs, consumption of alcohol is contraindicated (Olin et al., 1993).

Many drugs are included in this category. Among the various agents, differences exist not only in the duration of action, frequency of dosing, and side effects but also in the efficacy in treating a variety of conditions. Table 5-5 lists the most common NSAIDs.

ADJUNCTIVE ANALGESIC TREATMENTS

Another type of medication offers promise as an adjunct to analgesics. Utilizing tricyclic and heterocyclic (second generation) antidepressants as supplemental

Table 5-5 Nonsteroidal Anti-Inflammatory Drugs (NSAIDs)

Trade Name	Generic Name	Trade Name	Generic Name
Advil	Ibuprofen	Nalfon	Fenoprofen
Anaprox	Naproxen	Naprosyn	Naproxen
Ansaid	Flurbiprofen	Orudis	Ketoprofen
Clinoril	Sulindac	Ponstel	Mefenamic acid
Feldene	Piroxicam	Relafen	Nabumetone
Indocin	Indomethacin	Telectin	Tolmetin
Lodine	Etodolac	Toradol	Ketorolac
Meclomen	Meclofenamate	Voltaren	Diclofenac
Motrin	Ibuprofen		

medication in chronic pain conditions appears to be beneficial. These antidepressant analgesic effects operate by inhibiting the reuptake of neurotransmitter serotonin and norepinephrine. Increased serotonergic activity is associated with a rise in the pain threshold, while lowered serotonergic activity lowers the pain threshold (Trimble, 1990).

Chronic pain conditions for which antidepressants may be useful are migraine headaches, chronic tension headaches, diabetic neuropathy, tic douloureux, cancer pain, peripheral neuropathy with pain, postherpetic neuralgia, and arthritic pain. Tricyclics that may be prescribed for chronic pain include the following:

Trade Name	Generic Name	Dose
Adapin	Doxepin	50–300mg per day
Elavil	Amitriptyline	50–100mg per day
Endep	Amitriptyline	50–100mg per day
Sinequan	Doxepin	50–300mg per day
Tofranil	Imipramine	75–150mg per day [Olin et al., 1993]

Drugs prescribed for migraine headaches include the following:

Trade Name	Generic Name
Blocadren	Timolol
Ergostat	Ergotamine (a sublingual tablet)
Inderal	Propanolol
Medihaler Ergotamine	Ergotamine (an inhaler)
Sansert	Methysergide [Olin et al., 1993]

NARCOTIC ABUSE AND TOXICITY

A characteristic feature of all opioid or truly narcotic drugs is their potential for development of drug tolerance, psychological and physical dependence, and addiction. Because of the propensity for narcotic use to transform into drug abuse, these drugs are carefully monitored by the U.S. Drug Enforcement Administration (DEA). By providing stringent guidelines to pharmaceutical companies, doctors, nurses, and pharmacists, the DEA closely monitors distribution, dispensing, and administration of these drugs.

Unfortunately, illicit narcotic usage patterns are common. In the scope of their practices, physicians and pharmacists are liable to ensure that abusive patterns of narcotic usage do not develop. Situations of abuse often evolve when patients are under the care of more than one doctor, creating a situation where physicians are unaware of the drugs other doctors prescribe for their patients. If the patient patronizes only one drugstore and that store maintains a patient profile system, the pharmacist can easily detect excessive narcotic prescribing. However, the patient may be patronizing many different pharmacies, establishing a predicament in which neither the attending druggists nor the doctors have accurate information regarding the amount of narcotics the patient has been prescribed. For these reasons, it is imperative that counselors gather as much information as possible about their patients' drug prescriptions and drug intake. Measures to create statewide and national data bases that monitor prescription drug use have been resisted politically under the umbrella of the right to privacy.

Warnings associated with narcotic use are numerous. The dangerous depressant effects of opioid drugs are potentiated by the intake of other CNS depressants such as alcohol, barbiturates, benzodiazepines, or other sedative-hypnotic agents. The possibilities for lethal combinations of narcotics with other depressants are abundant. In such cases, the cause of death is usually respiratory depression and failure. Signs of opioid toxicity include respiratory depression, extreme somnolence, skeletal muscle flaccidity, and cold clammy skin (Olin et al., 1993). Opioid antagonists (Narcan, for example) have an excellent record for reversing the effects of narcotics overdose. Those suspected of narcotics overdose should be viewed as medical emergencies.

APPENDIX A

THE CENTRAL NERVOUS SYSTEM (CNS)

A three-layered covering called the **meninges** encapsulates the central nervous system, the spinal cord, and the brain (Carlson, 1991). Important brain structures include the cerebral cortex, the hypothalamus, the thalamus, the cerebellum, the reticular formation, the pons, and the medulla.

The cerebral cortex is the outer layer of the forebrain and is the most sophisticated part of the brain. It is often called the "gray matter" because the numerous cell bodies in this area have a grayish-brown appearance. Under the gray matter lie millions of myelinated axons that have a white appearance, and this area is referred to as "white matter." The cerebral cortex is divided front to back into the right and left hemispheres. The *corpus callosum* is the main group of axons or brain tissue that connects the right hemisphere with the left hemisphere. Each cerebral hemisphere has four areas or lobes, and each lobe has a specific function:

- Frontal lobe—planning and movement
- Parietal lobe—sensory stimulation
- Occipital lobe—vision
- Temporal lobe—hearing and memory

The *hypothalamus* is a collection of nuclei, which are groups of neuron cell bodies located inside the CNS. The hypothalamus controls the autonomic nervous system (ANS), the endocrine system, and organizes survival behavior (fighting, feeding, fleeing, and mating) for the species. The hypothalamus produces hormones that travel to the nearby anterior pituitary gland. This gland is referred to as the body's "master gland" because it controls other glandular secretions, such as sex and growth hormones. The hypothalamic hormones stimulate secretion of hormones from the anterior pituitary gland.

The *thalamus* is a large two-lobed structure located in the center of the brain. The thalamus receives information from sensory systems and relays messages to various areas in the brain. The thalamus is informally referred to as the "Grand Central Station" of the CNS.

The *cerebellum* is a distinct brain structure that is connected to the back of the brain stem. The cerebellum functions in coordination of movement, maintenance of equilibrium, and regulation of muscle tone.

The *reticular formation* is a structure in the core of the brain stem. It is important for controlling alertness, waking, sleeping, muscle tone, and various reflexes.

The *pons* is a part of the brain stem and includes part of the reticular formation. The pons plays an important role in sleep and arousal.

The *medulla* (or medulla oblongata) is also a component of the brain stem. It controls vital functions such as regulating the cardiovascular system, regulating respiration, skeletal muscle tone. It is located at the top of the spinal cord.

SYSTEMS THAT ENCOMPASS NUMEROUS AREAS OF THE BRAIN

The *reticular activating system* (RAS) extends from the central core of the brain stem to the cortex. The RAS is essential in initiating and maintaining wakefulness, introspection, and directing attention. Various tranquilizing drugs, benzodiazepines such as Valium, for example, suppress the RAS. Several stimulant drugs, such as amphetamines, activate the RAS. Continuous stimulation or intermittent overstimulation can lead to a wide range of psychiatric difficulties including anxiety, panic, and, finally, paranoia.

Pyramidal tracts are the main motor neuron tracts of the body. They originate in the cerebral cortex and cross over in the medulla. These nerve tracts are responsible for conducting the motor impulses from one side of the brain to the skeletal muscles on the opposite side of the body.

Extrapyramidal tracts, much more complex than pyramidal tracts, function to conduct impulses needed for muscle tone and equilibrium. Drugs that are said to produce **extrapyramidal symptoms** usually impair fine muscle coordination and balance and produce stereotypic, repetitive facial, tongue, and hand muscle twitches.

The *brain stem* is located at the base of the brain or the top of the spinal cord. The brain stem has three basic functions: (a) to relay messages to and from the cerebrum, cerebellum, and spinal cord; (b) as a component in various CNS activities such as the sleep–wake cycle, consciousness, and respiratory and cardiovascular control; and (c) to facilitate activities of the cranial nerves. Most of the 12 cranial nerves' cell bodies originate in the brain stem. Three prominent CNS structures, the medulla, the pons, and the midbrain, make up the brain stem.

The limbic system is a group of interconnected structures located underneath the cerebral cortex. Some of the important structures are the amygdala and hippocampus. The limbic system also connects to the hypothalamus and septal area of the brain. The limbic system is active in motivation, emotions, and in other processes.

THE PERIPHERAL NERVOUS SYSTEM

Communication between the CNS (brain and spinal cord) and the rest of the body is accomplished via spinal nerves and cranial nerves. The peripheral nervous system (PNS) is comprised of all the nervous tissue outside the CNS, including the 12 cranial nerves and 31 spinal nerves.

Cranial nerves consist of 12 pairs of nerves that mostly serve the sensory and motor functions in the head and neck region. Special names are given to each pair of nerves, with the name of the nerve suggesting its function.

Spinal nerves are the collection of 31 nerve pairs that branch out from the front and back of the spinal cord. No special names are assigned to the spinal nerves. Each set of nerves is represented by a number that corresponds to the level of the spinal column on which the nerve pair originates. There are eight cervical, 12 thoracic, five lumbar, and five sacral pairs, and one coccygeal pair of spinal nerves. Nerve fibers that carry messages or commands from the spinal cord to organs, muscles, or glands are called *efferent fibers* or axons. Sensory information perceived is relayed to the spinal cord along *afferent fibers* or axons.

The PNS is made up of two major divisions. The **somatic nervous system** receives information from sensory neurons and controls skeletal movement. The **autonomic nervous system** (ANS) is sometimes referred to as the involuntary nervous system.

The ANS functions to regulate smooth muscle, cardiac muscle, and glands; it governs actions of various organ systems (stomach, pancreas, intestines, lungs, bladder, sweat glands, salivary glands, skin, sex organs, and more). ANS has two major divisions, the **parasympathetic nervous system** and the **sympathetic nervous system**. Both systems innervate nerves to most organs. The parasympathetic nervous system controls "feed and breed" activities during times of relaxation, producing a decrease in heart rate and an increase in digestive activity. The parasympathetic system also facilitates activities that increase the body's supply of stored energy. The sympathetic nervous system is activated in times of excitement and exertion known to produce the body's "fight or flight" responses. It mobilizes energy, increases blood flow to vital skeletal muscles, stimulates the release of adrenalin, and increases heart rate and the level of sugar in the blood.

APPENDIX B

PHARMACOKINETICS

The term **pharmacokinetics** refers to the study of in vivo (occurring inside the body) drug processes and includes administration and absorption, distribution, metabolism, and excretion.

ADMINISTRATION AND ABSORPTION

Various methods are available for administering drugs. The rate of absorption is regulated by the method of administration, so the choice of method is an important variable in drug therapy. Drugs that are given intermittently are administered according to specific schedules. Box B-1 lists common intermittent dosing schedules.

ORAL DRUG ADMINISTRATION

Oral drug forms include liquids, tablets, and capsules. Liquid dosage forms have the fastest absorption rate. Tablets are absorbed more slowly. Capsules are often formulated as time-release or sustained-release products, with the advantage of requiring fewer daily doses. A variety of problems may occur with oral drug administration.

Box B-1 Dosing Schedules for Administration of Drugs

Abbreviations used in patient charts to represent common intermittent dosing schedules are:

qid (4 times a day)	**qd** (every day)
tid (3 times a day)	**hs** (at bedtime)
bid (2 times a day)	**am** (in the morning)
ac (before meals)	**pm** (in the evening)
pc (after meals)	

With intermittent dosing, drug levels in the blood will fluctuate. Continuous methods of administering drugs avoid shifts in drug levels. A continuous intravenous method of administration prevents fluctuating drug levels in the blood.

Oral administration is the slowest method of absorption, and the onset of a drug's effect is less predictable because drug absorption from the gastrointestinal tract is often erratic. Variables that affect the rate of absorption of a drug are related to the concomitant intake of food and the drug's pH (acidity or basicity) relative to the pH values of the stomach and the intestines. Drugs can exist in two interconvertible forms, a water-soluble or ionized form and a lipid-soluble or nonionized form. A drug's lipid-to-water solubility is determined by the pH of the drug relative to the pH of the body fluid that harbors the drug.

Drugs administered orally undergo what is called *first-pass metabolism*. First-pass metabolism occurs immediately after the drug is absorbed from the gastrointestinal tract. The blood carries the drug to the liver, where some of the drug is metabolized, which renders the drug inactive or unable to exert its desired effect.

INJECTABLE DRUGS

Three basic methods are used for injecting medication: intravenous, intramuscular, and subcutaneous injections.

Intravenous (into the vein) injection has the fastest absorption rate. Because of this, it is potentially the most dangerous form of injection.

Intramuscular (into the muscle) injection provides a means for rapid absorption but is not as fast as intravenous injection.

Subcutaneous (under a layer of skin) injection is used when a slower and more constant rate of absorption is recommended.

Some injectable antipsychotics are formulated to prolong the effects of the drug. Two examples are *Haldol Decanoate* and *Prolixin Decanoate*. Effects of both injectable drugs can last three to four weeks. These two drugs can be used in schizophrenic patients who are noncompliant in taking medication (Olin et al., 1993; Ponterotto, 1985).

OTHER METHODS

A variety of other methods can be used for administering drugs. These include *sublingual* (a tablet placed under the tongue), *buccal* (drug positioned between cheek and gum), *vaginal, anal*, and *oral* or *nasal inhalation*. In each of these alternate administration methods, a drug is readily absorbed into the bloodstream because of the highly vascular membranes in each of these areas.

DISTRIBUTION

Once administered and absorbed in the bloodstream, drugs are carried to various body tissues via the circulatory system. Blood capillaries deliver drugs to different areas in the body. For most drugs, capillary pores are large enough to allow free passage to the outside.

PROTEIN BINDING

Some drugs bind irreversibly to circulating plasma proteins. A protein-bound drug is usually so large that it is unable to exit the capillary, rendering it inactive in the bloodstream until separation from the protein. Drug protein binding also hinders a drug's metabolism and excretion, thus causing a drug to remain in the body longer, which increases the drug's half-life. The term **half-life** is used to describe the average time required to eliminate one-half of a drug's dose. Theoretically, about six half-lives are needed to remove almost all of any given drug. Therefore, if a drug has a half-life of four hours, after 24 hours (six half-lives times four-hour half-life) nearly all the drug will be excreted. Drugs with short half-lives require a more frequent dosing schedule than drugs with long half-lives.

LIPID SOLUBILITY

Passage across various membranes or barriers in the body, such as the stomach, intestines, blood-brain barrier (BBB), and placenta, depends on a drug's lipid (fat) solubility. Drugs with a high lipid solubility cross the BBB easily and remain in the brain tissues longer than water-soluble drugs do. This difference is explained by the fact that lipid-soluble chemicals or drugs are stored in the body's fat tissue.

METABOLISM

Most drugs are metabolized or broken down by liver enzymes, which act to transform chemicals or drugs into more water-soluble or hydrophilic entities so the drugs can be excreted in the urine. Because of the decline in liver activity among the elderly, it takes them longer to metabolize drugs. Therefore, drug dosages for the geriatric population are usually reduced.

EXCRETION

The kidney is the body's main excretory organ. Less frequently, drugs are eliminated from the body via the lungs, sweat glands, saliva, feces, bile, and breast milk.

SIDE EFFECTS, INTERACTIONS, AND TOXICITY

SIDE EFFECTS

Other terms used to describe drug side effects are *adverse reactions and untoward or unwanted effects.* Rather than being selectively carried to a specific or targeted area, drugs are widely distributed throughout the body. Therefore, a drug will bind with any receptor that its chemical structure will allow. This nonselective drug binding capacity explains the origin of drug side effects. Adverse drug side effects must be monitored, and a drug's benefits should outweigh any detrimental side effects. Generally, as the dosage is increased, symptoms of the disease decrease but side effects increase. Physicians try to determine the best drug dose to alleviate disease symptoms with the least number of side effects.

Another common method used to decrease or lessen side effects of a drug is to have **drug holidays**, blocks of time when the drug is not administered.

A **drug allergy** is different from side effects of a drug. An allergy involves histamine reaction. Any amount of the drug can elicit an allergic response. Therefore, a dosage reduction will not prevent an allergic reaction. Allergic reactions can range from mild to severe and are sometimes fatal.

DRUG INTERACTIONS

Factors that contribute to drug interactions include **protein binding** and **enzyme induction** or **inhibition.**

PROTEIN BINDING. Two drugs can compete for binding sites on circulating plasma proteins. Initiating therapy with drug B, which has a high affinity for protein binding, can displace drug A, which is already bound to plasma proteins. This type of drug interaction can be dangerous because of the possibility that toxic blood levels of released drug A may result.

ENZYME INDUCTION OR INHIBITION. One drug can accelerate the metabolism of another drug by inducing or activating liver enzymes that mediate a drug's metabolism. Conversely, inhibition of hepatic (liver) enzymes by one drug can increase the drug level in the blood and, in turn, increase the pharmacological activity of another drug.

TOXICITY

A drug or specific drug dosage is said to be *toxic* when it damages the brain or other vital organs in the body. Some drugs are toxic at low dosages; other drugs require a larger dosage to inflict brain or organ damage. When a drug requires only a small amount to produce its desired effects, this drug is said to have a low therapeutic dose. If this same drug, with the low therapeutic dose, also has a high toxic dose, the drug is described as having a large or wide **therapeutic window**. A therapeutic window is the range of dosages wherein a drug is both safe and effective.

Glossary

Acetylcholine (ACh) One of the major neurotransmitters, located both in the central and peripheral nervous systems. ACh plays an excitatory role in processes involving memory, mood, learning, attention, muscular contraction, and sleep.

Action potential (AP) A change in a nerve's electrical charge to the extent that the nerve is stimulated.

Acute pain Pain, due to disease or injury, that lasts less than 30 days and that is functional in restricting movement of the person or injured area.

Adrenalin A neural transmitter produced by the adrenal gland, exerting most of its effect in the peripheral nervous system, where it functions to maintain heart rate and blood pressure. Also referred to as *epinephrine.*

Agonist A drug or chemical that increases the availability for action or mimics the action of an endogenous neurotransmitter.

Akathisia A physical state of nervousness that is characterized by compulsion to move or in which an individual is in constant motion.

Akinesia A complete or partial loss of muscular movement.

Amino acids A group of organic compounds used as the building blocks of proteins. Some also act as neurotransmitters.

Antagonist A drug that decreases the availability or action of a neurotransmitter.

Anticholinergic properties The properties of drugs that block the action of the neurotransmitter acetylcholine. Side effects include dry mouth, constipation, blurred near vision, urinary retention, increased heart rate, and delayed ejaculation.

Anxiolytic An agent that reduces anxiety. Also referred to as a *minor tranquilizer.*

Ataxia Lack of muscular coordination.

Autonomic nervous system (ANS) A branch of the nervous system that is concerned with involuntary control in the body. The ANS has two major divisions, the parasympathetic nervous system and the sympathetic nervous system.

Axon Part of a neuron, generally shaped like a long, slender tube, that relays impulses from the soma (cell body of the neuron) to the terminal buttons of the neuron.

Barbiturates A class of central nervous system–depressant drugs that were once frequently prescribed as sedatives.

Benzodiazepines (BDZs) A group of structurally related compounds that have sedative properties. Because of their greater safety margin, BDZs have, for the most part, replaced the barbiturates, a more dangerous class of sedatives.

Beta–blockers or beta-adrenergic blocking agents A group of structurally related drugs used to treat hypertension, migraines, a variety of heart problems, and other problems.

Biological amine hypothesis of depression The view that functional deficits in the brain of the catecholamine NT norepinephrine or the indoleamine NT serotonin—or both—cause depression.

Blood-brain barrier (BBB) A barrier in the central nervous system that exists between circulating blood in the brain and the fluid that surrounds the brain tissue.

Bruxism Teeth grinding while sleeping.

Catecholamines A class of neurotransmitters derived from the compound catechol. Each neurotransmitter in this group has an amine group. Neurotransmitters in this class are dopamine, norepinephrine, and epinephrine.

Chronic pain Pain that evolves into a prolonged or long-term episodic condition of more than three months and that can no longer be directly attributed to continuing tissue damage.

Convergence of information The gathering of information from many other neurons by dendrites.

Delirium A state of clouded consciousness in which an individual is unable to focus or sustain attention. Perceptual disturbances (hallucination and illusions), sleep and affective disturbances, disorientation, and memory impairment are all components of delirium.

Delta waves The deep restorative sleep in the human sleep cycle.

Dementia A loss of intellectual ability that results in impairment in occupational and social functioning.

Dendrite A part of the neuron that branches off toward other nerve cells. Dendrites contain receptors, which receive messages from other nerve cells.

Depolarization A process that occurs when a neuron becomes more positive, producing an excitatory effect. Also referred to as *excitatory postsynaptic potential (EPSP)*.

Diuretic An agent that increases the amount of urine the kidney excretes.

Divergence of information The dispersal of information by axons to many other neurons.

Dopamine (DA) A neurotransmitter that produces both excitatory and inhibitory effects in the central nervous system. Dopamine is involved in movement, learning and attention, Parkinson's disease, and schizophrenia.

Dopamine hypothesis of schizophrenia The view that either functional changes in the catecholamine NT dopamine in the brain or an excess of dopamine causes schizophrenia.

Double depression A state that occurs when individuals with dysthymia also experience an episode of major depression.

Drug allergy A situation wherein any amount of a particular drug introduced into the body elicits an allergic response.

Drug holiday A period of time when a routinely prescribed drug is deliberately not administered.

Dynorphins An endogenous group of opioid neurotransmitters that have analgesic effects.

Dyskinesia   Side effects of antipsychotic drugs. Dyskinesia is characterized as inappropriate movements (spasms, tics, and involuntary movements).

Dyssomnias   A group of sleep disorders with the chief problem being amount, quality, or timing of sleep.

Dysthymia   Depressive neurosis marked by either long-term depression or chronic, but sub-acute depression.

Dystonic reactions   Side effects of antipsychotic drugs. Dystonic reactions are characterized by involuntary and inappropriate postures.

Electroencephalogram (EEG)   The polygraphic recording of the brain's electrical activity (brain waves).

Endocytosis   The process through which neurotransmitters are reuptaken.

Endorphins   Endogenous neurotransmitters that have an analgesic effect similar to morphine. Also referred to as *opioid peptides.*

Enkephalins   An endogenous group of opioid neurotransmitters with analgesic effects.

Enzymatic deactivation   A degradation process of a neurotransmitter by an enzyme.

Enzyme   Organic compounds in living cells. Enzymes act as catalysts for a variety of the body's chemical reactions.

Enzyme induction   The process by which the liver is induced to manufacture higher levels of enzymes to break down either naturally occurring body chemicals or exogenous drugs.

Epinephrine (Epi)   A neurotransmitter produced by the adrenal gland. Epinephrine exerts most of its effect in the peripheral nervous system, where it functions to maintain heart rate and blood pressure. Also referred to as *adrenalin.*

Excitatory postsynaptic potential (EPSP)   A process that occurs when a neuron becomes more positive, producing an excitatory effect. Also referred to as *depolarization.*

Exocytosis   The process of a neuron releasing neurotransmitters into the synapse.

Extrapyramidal symptoms   A group of side effects commonly associated with antipsychotic medications. Extrapyramidal symptoms include Parkinsonian symptoms, dystonic reaction, tardive dyskinesia, dyskinesia, and akathisia.

Functional disorder   A general term applied to a condition when reasons for change in function are not apparent.

Functional psychoses   Abnormal behaviors that cannot be attributed to any single known cause.

Galactorrhea   Abnormal flow of breast milk or lactation.

Gamma-aminobutyric acid (GABA)   An inhibitory neurotransmitter found in the brain.

Glial cells   Support cells, found in the nervous system, that function in various ways.

Glutamate   An excitatory neurotransmitter that lowers the threshold for neural excitation.

Glycine   A neurotransmitter that has inhibitory effects in the spinal cord.

Gynecomastia   A condition of abnormally large mammary glands in males (milk may be secreted).

Half-life   The average time required to eliminate one-half of a drug's dose.

Heterocyclic antidepressants   A broad class of antidepressant drugs developed and introduced after tricyclic antidepressants often called *second generation antidepressants.*

Hirsutism   Abnormal hair growth.

Hyperpolarization   A process whereby a neuron's electrical charge becomes more negative, causing an inhibitory or stabilizing effect on the neuron. Also called *inhibitory postsynaptic potential (IPSP)*.

Hypnotic A drug capable of inducing a state of central nervous system depression that resembles normal sleep.

Hypoglycemic agent A drug with the ability to lower the body's blood sugar level.

Hypomania A state of mild mania and excitement with modest behavioral change.

Idiosyncratic reaction A side effect that occurs in only a very small percentage of the population.

Inhibitory postsynaptic potential (IPSP) A process whereby a neuron's electrical charge becomes more negative, causing an inhibitory or stabilizing effect on the neuron. Also called *hyperpolarization*.

Insomnia A perceived decrease in the quality or quantity of sleep, which affects the individual's daytime functioning.

Ions Small, electrically charged molecules.

Lipid A fat or fat-like substance.

Lipophilic molecules Molecules that dissolve readily in fats. *Lipophilic* is a term used to describe a substance's (or drug's) affinity for fats.

Lysergic acid diethylamide (LSD) A psychedelic drug that is similar in structure to the neurotransmitter serotonin.

Major tranquilizer Another term for antipsychotic drugs.

Meninges A three-layered covering that encapsulates the central nervous system (brain and spinal cord).

Minor tranquilizer An agent that reduces anxiety. Also referred to as an *anxiolytic*.

Monoamine oxidase inhibitor antidepressants (MAOIs) A group of antidepressant agents that exert their desired effect by inhibiting the enzyme monoamine oxidase, which is normally responsible for the degradation of monoamine neurotransmitters.

Monoamines A class of neurotransmitters. Each neurotransmitter in this group has a single amine group as part of its chemical structure. Neurotransmitters in this class include dopamine, norepinephrine, epinephrine, and serotonin.

Myelin sheath A protective covering of axons. The myelin sheath also improves distance conduction.

Narcolepsy A sleep disorder characterized by excessive daytime sleepiness, falling asleep at inappropriate times, cataplexy, sleep paralysis, and hypnogogic hallucinations.

Neuralgia A condition of severe, sharp nerve pain.

Neuroleptic Phenothiazine drugs and Haldol. Neuroleptics are used to treat the positive symptoms of schizophrenia.

Neuroleptic malignant syndrome A very severe, potentially life-threatening complication that can occur when using antipsychotic drugs. The syndrome is characterized by catatonia, unstable blood pressure, unstable heart rate, hyperthermia, mutism, and stupor.

Neuroleptic state A state induced in schizophrenics when treated with antipsychotic drugs. A neuroleptic state is characterized by psychomotor slowing, emotional quieting, and affective indifference.

Neuromodulators (NMs) Chemicals that facilitate communication between neurons.

Neuron A highly specialized nerve cell that conducts impulses throughout the brain and body.

Neuropeptides Chains of amino acids that either act on their own or act to enhance or inhibit the effects of other neurotransmitters.

Neuropharmacology The study of drugs' effects on the nervous system.

Neurotransmission Communication between neurons.

Neurotransmitters (NTs) Chemicals that facilitate communication between neurons.

Nightmares Dreams with anxiety-provoking content. Nightmares are often open to recall and occur during REM sleep.

Night terrors A sleep disorder characterized by extreme vocalizations, sweating, or fast heart rate.

Nociceptor A pain receptor located in the skin.

Norepinephrine (NE) An excitatory neurotransmitter involved with emotions and with maintaining wakefulness and alertness.

Opiate A naturally occurring or synthetic analgesic agent that mimics the effects of morphine.

Opioid peptides Endogenous neuropeptide analgesic agents. Also referred to as *endorphins*.

Opioids Another term for *opiates* or narcotic analgesics.

Opponent process A situation in which excitatory and inhibitory neurotransmitter systems counteract each other to have a balancing effect.

Organic brain syndrome A term used to describe an assortment of conditions characterized by impaired brain functioning without indicating the etiology of the impairment.

Organic psychoses Psychotic behavior that results from insult or trauma to the brain.

Parasomnias A group of sleep disorders characterized by an abnormal event during sleep.

Parasympathetic nervous system A division of the autonomic nervous system that is active during times of relaxation.

Parkinsonian effects or symptoms Side effects that resemble symptoms of Parkinson's disease. They are common in antipsychotic drug therapy.

Parkinson's disease A chronic progressive disease characterized by rigidity, tremors, and muscle weakness resulting from an imbalance of dopamine and acetylcholine in the brain.

Pharmacokinetics The study of in vivo drug processes, including administration, absorption, distribution, metabolism, and excretion.

Pharmacopsychologist A psychologist trained as an expert in psychoactive medications who may or may not have prescription privileges.

Pharmacopsychology The study of psychoactive medications. Also referred to as *psychopharmacology*.

Phenothiazines The oldest class of antipsychotic drugs. All have a similar chemical structure.

Polydipsia Excessive thirst.

Polypharmacy Condition of being treated with an excessive number of prescription drugs.

Polyuria Excessive urination.

PRN In drug therapy, PRN (*pro re nata*), refers to medication given on demand or as needed.

Prophylactic treatment Drug therapy used to prevent the onset or recurrence of a disease.

Protein binding The ability of a drug to attach to proteins circulating in the bloodstream.

Psychotoxic Drugs that alter central nervous system functioning. Also referred to as *psychotropic*.

Psychotropic Drugs that alter central nervous system functioning. Also referred to as *psychotoxic.*

Rapid eye movement (REM) sleep One of the sleep stages characterized by regular, fast eye movements; muscle paralysis; and occurrence of dream activity.

Rebound hyperexcitability A state of rapid rise of neural excitation due to abrupt discontinuation of tranquilizing drugs.

Receptor Specialized molecules on neurons that are targets for specific neurotransmitters.

Reuptake The process of extremely rapid removal of the neurotransmitter from the synaptic cleft.

Second generation antidepressants A group of newer antidepressants that are less toxic and have fewer side effects than the older tricyclic antidepressants.

Serotonin (5-HT) A neurotransmitter involved in the inhibition of activity and behavior. It is active in mood regulation; control of eating, sleeping, and arousal; and pain regulation.

Signal anxieties Anxieties that signal (result from) unresolved psychodynamic conflicts and that usually do not remit until underlying issues are resolved.

Sleep apnea A sleep disorder characterized by cessations in breathing interfering with the quality of sleep.

Soma The cell body of the neuron. The soma holds the nucleus and gives rise to the axon.

Somatic nervous system One of the two main divisions of the peripheral nervous system. The somatic nervous system is active in receiving information for sensory neurons and controlling skeletal movement.

Somnambulism Sleepwalking.

Steroid psychosis Psychotic behavior precipitated by the use of corticosteroids.

Stress-diathesis model Stress in the environment interacting with an individual's genetic predisposition to trigger the onset of an illness.

Substance P A neurotransmitter released in the spinal cord to facilitate relaying pain messages.

Sympathetic nervous system One of the divisions of the autonomic nervous system that is activated in times of excitement or stress.

Synapse The point where two neurons meet and relay information.

Synaptic cleft or gap The area between two adjacent neurons in which neurotransmitters travel.

Tardive dyskinesia A late-appearing side effect of antipsychotic drugs. Tardive dyskinesia is characterized by abnormal, involuntary movements of the mouth, face, limbs, and trunk.

Teratogenic effects Development of a severely abnormal or deformed fetus due to the mother's ingestion of drugs during pregnancy.

Terminal buttons Knob-like structure, located on the end of a neuron's axon, where neurotransmitters are stored.

Therapeutic window The range in which a drug's doses are both safe and effective. A wide therapeutic window or margin indicates that a drug's therapeutic dose is much lower than its toxic dose.

Tricyclic antidepressants (TCAs) A class of antidepressants with the same basic three-ring chemical structure. Tricyclic agents are notorious for their bothersome side effects.

Vesicle A small sac inside a neuron's terminal button that contains the neurotransmitter.

References

ABRAMOWICZ, M. (Ed.). (1990, January 16). Drugs that cause psychiatric symptoms. *The Medical Letter, 31,* 113–118.

ALLEBECK, P. (1989). Schizophrenia: A life-shortening disease. *Schizophrenia Bulletin, 15,* 81–89.

ALTMAIER, E. M., & JOHNSON, B. D. (1992). Health-related applications of counseling psychology: Toward health promotion and disease prevention across the life span. In S. Brown & R. Lent (Eds.), *Handbook of counseling psychology* (2nd ed., pp. 315–348). New York: Wiley.

AMERICAN MEDICAL ASSOCIATION. (1983). Antipsychotic drugs. In *AMA drug evaluations.* Philadelphia: Saunders.

AMERICAN PSYCHIATRIC ASSOCIATION. (1994). *Diagnostic and statistical manual of mental disorders (4th ed.).* Washington, DC: American Psychiatric Association.

ANDREASEN, N. C. (1989). The American concept of schizophrenia. *Schizophrenia Bulletin, 15*(4), 519–531.

ANGERMEYER, M. C., KUHN, L., & GOLDSTEIN, J. M. (1990). Gender and the course of schizophrenia: Differences in treated outcomes. *Schizophrenia Bulletin, 16*(2), 293–305.

BALDESSARINI, R. J. (1985). Drugs and the treatment of psychiatric disorders. In A. G. Gilman, L. S. Goodman, T. W. Rall, & F. Murad (Eds.), *The pharmacological basis of therapeutics* (7th ed., pp. 387–445). New York: Macmillan.

BALDESSARINI, R. J. (1993). Drugs and the treatment of psychiatric disorders. In A. G. Gilman, T. W. Rall, A. S. Nies, & P. Taylor (Eds.), *The pharmacological basis of therapeutics* (8th ed., pp. 383–435). New York: McGraw-Hill.

BARLOW, D. H. (1988). *Anxiety and its disorders: The nature and treatment of anxiety and panic.* New York: Guilford Press.

BARLOW, D. H., & CERNY, J. A. (1988). *Psychological treatment of panic.* New York: Guilford Press.

BARON, M., GRUEN, R., RAINER, J. D., KANE, J., ASNIS, L., & LORD, S. (1985). A family study of schizophrenia and normal control probands: Implications for the spectrum concept of schizophrenia. *American Journal of Psychiatry, 142*(4), 447–455.

BEASLEY, C. M., DORNSEIF, B., BOSOMWORTH, J., SAYLER, M., RAMPEY, A., HEILIGENSTEIN, J., THOMPSON, V., MURPHY, D., & MASICA, D. (1991). Fluoxetine and suicide: A meta-analysis of controlled trials of treatment for depression. *BMJ, 303,* 685–692.

BEASLEY, C. M., MASICA, D., & POTVIN, J. (1992). Fluoxetine: A review of receptor and functional effects and their clinical implication. *Psychopharmacology, 107,* 1–10.

BECK, A. T., & EMERY, G. (1985). *Anxiety disorders and phobias: A cognitive perspective.* New York: Basic Books.

BECK, A. T., RUSH, A. J., SHAW, B. F., & EMERY, G. (1979). *The cognitive therapy of depression.* New York: Guilford Press.

BEDDER, M. D., SOIFER, P. E., & MULHALL, J. J. V. (1991). A comparison of patient-controlled analgesia and bolus PRN intravenous morphine in the intensive care environment. *Clinical Journal of Pain, 7*(3), 205–208.

BELLACK, A. S. (1989). A comprehensive model for treatment of schizophrenia. In A. S. Bellack (Ed.), *A clinical guide for the treatment of schizophrenia* (pp. 1–22). New York: Plenum.

BERNTZEN, D., & GOTESTAM, K. G. (1987). Effects of on-demand versus fixed-interval schedule in the treatment of chronic pain with analgesic compounds. *Journal of Consulting and Clinical Psychology, 55*(2), 213–217.

BRANCONNIER, R. J., COLE, J. O., GHAZVINIAN, S., SPERA, K., OXENKRUG, G. F., & BASS, J. L. (1983). Clinical pharmacology of bupropion and imipramine in elderly depressives. *The Journal of Clinical Psychiatry, 44*(5), 130–134.

BRENNER, H. D., DENCKER, S. J., GOLDSTEIN, M. J., HUBBARD, J. W., KEEGAN, D. L., KRUGER, G., KULHANEK, F., LIBERMAN, R. P., MALM, U., & MIDHA, K. K. (1990). Defining treatment refractoriness in schizophrenia. *Schizophrenia Bulletin, 16*(4), 551–561.

BROWN, J. H. (1993). Atropine, scopolamine, and related antimuscarinic drugs. In A. G. Gilman, T. W. Rall, A. S. Nies, & P. Taylor (Eds.), *The pharmacological basis of therapeutics* (8th ed., pp. 150–165). New York: McGraw-Hill.

BROWN, W. A., & HERZ, L. R. (1989). Response to neuroleptic drugs as a device for classifying schizophrenia. *Schizophrenia Bulletin, 15*(1), 123–128.

BUSSE, E., & SIMPSON, D. (1983). Depression and antidepressants and the elderly. *The Journal of Clinical Psychiatry, 44*(5), 35–40.

CARLSON, N. R. (1991). *Physiology of behavior* (4th ed.). Boston: Allyn & Bacon.

CAROFF, S. N., & MANN, S. C. (1988). Neuroleptic malignant syndrome. *Psychopharmacology Bulletin, 24*(1), 25–29.

CHAFETZ, M. D., & BUELOW, G. D. (in press). A training model for psychologists with prescription privilege: Clinical pharmacopsychologists. *Professional Psychology: Research and Practice.*

CHARNEY, D. S., HENINGER, G. R., & BREIER, A. (1984). Noradrenergic function in panic anxiety: Effects of yohimbine in healthy subjects and patients with agoraphobia and panic disorder. *Archives of General Psychiatry, 41,* 751–763.

COOPER, J. R., BLOOM, F. E., & ROTH, R. H. (1991). *The biochemical basis of neuropharmacology.* New York: Oxford University Press.

COURSEY, R. D. (1989). Psychotherapy with persons suffering from schizophrenia: The need for a new agenda. *Schizophrenia Bulletin, 15*(3), 349–353.

CROOK, T. H., KUPFER, D. J., HOCH, C. C., & REYNOLDS, C. F. (1987). Treatment of sleep disorders in the elderly. In H. Meltzer (Ed.), *Psychopharmacology: The third generation of progress* (pp. 1159–1165). New York: Raven Press.

DAWKINS, K., & POTTER, W. (1991). Gender differences in pharmacokinetics and pharmacodynamics of psychotropics: Focus on women. *Psychopharmacology Bulletin, 27,* 417–423.

DEARDOFF, W. W., RUBIN, H. S., & SCOTT, D. W. (1991). Comprehensive multidisciplinary treatment of chronic pain: A follow-up study of treated & non-treated groups. *Pain, 45,* 35–43.

DELGADO, P. L., PRICE, L., MILLER, H., SALOMON, R., LICINIO, J., KRYSTAL, J., HENINGER, G., & CHARNEY, D. (1991). Rapid serotonin depletion as a provocative challenge test for patients with major depression: Relevance to antidepressant action and the neurobiology of depression. *Psychopharmacology Bulletin, 27,* 321–330.

DUGAS, J. E. (1987). Panic disorders: Pathophysiology and treatment. *Pharmacy Times, 53*(11), 120–131.

EGBERT, A. M. (1991). Help for the hurting elderly. *Post Graduate Medicine, 89*(4), 217–228.

FERRIS, R. M., COOPER, B. R., & MAXWELL, R. A. (1983). Studies of bupropion's mechanism of antidepressant activity. *The Journal of Clinical Psychiatry, 44*(5), 74–79.

FORDYCE, W. E., & STEGER, J. C. (1979). Chronic pain. In O. F. Pomerleau, & J. P. Brady (Eds.), *Behavioral medicine: Theory and practice* (pp. 125–153). Baltimore: Wilkins & Wilkins.

FREDRICK, J. F., & FREDRICK, N. J. (1985). The hospice experience: Possible effects in altering the biochemistry of bereavement. *The Hospice Journal, 1*(3), 81–90.

FULLER, S. H., & UNDERWOOD, E. S. (1989, August). Update on antidepressant medications. *U.S. Pharmacist*, pp. 35, 36, 39, 42, 44, 46.

GADOW, K. D. (1992). Pediatric psychopharmacotherapy: A review of recent research. *Journal of Child Psychology and Psychiatry, 33*, 153–195.

GARVEY, M. (1990). Benzodiazepines for panic disorder. *Postgraduate Medicine, 90*(5), 245–246, 249–252.

GILDERMAN, A. (1979). Drug-induced psychiatric illnesses. In Hoffman-LaRoche, Inc., *Psychopharmacology for practicing pharmacists*. Pamphlet. New Jersey: Nuttley.

GOODNICK, P. J. (1991). Pharmacokinetics of second generation antidepressants: Bupropion. *Psychopharmacology Bulletin, 27*, 516–519.

GOSSEL, T. A., & WUEST, J. R. (1992). Alzheimer's disease, part 1: Pathogenesis, symptoms and outcome. *Mississippi Pharmacist, 18*(4), 27–29.

GOVONI, L. E., & HAYES, J. E. (1985). *Drugs and nursing implication*. Connecticut: Appleton-Century-Crofts.

HAMMEN, C. L. (1991). Mood disorders. In M. Hersen & S. M. Turner (Eds.), *Adult psychopathology and diagnosis* (2nd ed.). New York: Wiley.

HAURI, P. J. (1985). Primary sleep disorders and insomnia. In T. L. Riley (Ed.), *Clinical aspects of sleep and sleep disturbances*. Boston: Butterworth.

HEINRICHS, D. W., & CARPENTER, W. T. (1985). Prospective study of prodromal symptoms in schizophrenic relapse. *American Journal of Psychiatry, 142*(3), 371–373.

HOFFMAN, B. B., & LEFKOWITZ, R. J. (1993). Catecholamines and sympathomimetic drugs. In A. G. Gilman, T. W. Rall, A. S. Nies, & P. Taylor (Eds.), *The pharmacological basis of therapeutics* (8th ed., pp. 221–243). New York: McGraw-Hill.

INSEL, P. A. (1993). Analgesics-antipyretics and anti-inflammatory agents: Drugs employed in the treatment of rheumatoid arthritis and gout. In A. G. Gilman, T. W. Rall, A. S. Nies, & P. Taylor (Eds.), *The pharmacological basis of therapeutics* (8th ed., pp. 638–681). New York: McGraw-Hill.

JAFFE, J. H., & MARTIN, W. R. (1985). Opioid analgesics and antagonists. In A. G. Gilman, L. S. Goodman, T. W. Rall, & F. Murad (Eds.), *The pharmacological basis of therapeutics* (7th ed., pp. 491–531). New York: Macmillan.

JAFFE, J. H., & MARTIN, W. R. (1993). Opioid analgesics and antagonists. In A. G. Gilman, T. W. Rall, A. S. Nies, & P. Taylor (Eds.), *The pharmacological basis of therapeutics* (8th ed., pp. 485–521). New York: McGraw-Hill.

JESTE, D. V., & WYATT, R. J. (1982) *Understanding and treating tardive dyskinesia*. New York: Guilford Press.

JOHNSON, D. A. (1989). Treatment of depression in schizophrenia. In B. Lerer & S. Gershon (Eds.), *New directions in affective disorders* (pp. 509–516). New York: Springer-Verlag.

JONAS, J. M., & SCHAUMBURG, R. (1991). *Everything you need to know about Prozac*. New York: Bantam.

JOYCE, P. R., & PAYKEL, E. S. (1989). Predictors of drug response in depression. *Archives of General Psychiatry, 46*(1), 89–99.

JULIEN, R. M. (1992). *A primer of drug action* (6th ed.). New York: W. H. Freeman.

KANE, J. M. (1989). Innovations in the psychopharmacologic treatment of schizophrenia. In A. S. Bellack (Ed.), *A clinical guide for the treatment of schizophrenia* (pp. 43–76). New York: Plenum.

KIMBERLY, A., ELLISON, J., SHERA, M., PRATT, L., LANGFORD, B., COLE, J., WHITE, K., LAVORI, P., & KELLER, M. (1992). Pharmacotherapy observed in a large prospective longitudinal study on anxiety disorders. *Psychopharmacology Bulletin, 28,* 131–137.

KLAASSEN, C. D. (1993). Nonmetallic environmental toxicants: Air pollutants, solvents and vapors, and pesticides. In A. G. Gilman, T. W. Rall, A. S. Nies, & P. Taylor (Eds.), *The pharmacological basis of therapeutics* (8th ed., pp. 1615–1639). New York: McGraw-Hill.

KLEIN, G. R. (1987). Pharmacotherapy of childhood hyperactivity: An update. In H. Y. Meltzer (Ed.), *Psychopharmacology: The third generation of progress* (pp. 1215–1224). New York: Raven Press.

LAWSON, G. W., & COPPERRIDER, C. A. (1988). *Clinical psychopharmacology.* Gaithersburg, MD: Aspen.

LECCESE, A. P. (1991). *Drugs and society.* Englewood Cliffs, NJ: Prentice Hall.

LICKEY, M. E., & GORDON, B. (1983). *Drugs for mental illness.* New York: Freeman.

LOEBEL, A. D., LIEBERMAN, J. A., ALVIR, J. M., MAYERHOFF, D. I., GEISLER, S. H., & SZYMANSKI, S. R. (1992). Duration of psychosis and outcome in first-episode schizophrenia. *American Journal of Psychiatry, 149*(9), 1183–1188.

MARDER, S. R., MINTZ, J., PUTTEN, T. V., LEBELL, M., WIRSHING, W. C., & JOHNSTON-CRONK, K. (1991). Early prediction of relapse in schizophrenia: An application of receiver operating characteristic (ROC) methods. *Psychopharmacology Bulletin, 27*(1), 79–82.

MAXMEN, J. C. (1991). *Psychotropic drugs fast facts.* New York: Norton.

MCBRIDE, P. A., ANDERSON, G., KHAIT, V., SUNDAY, S., & HALMI, K. (1991). Serotonergic responsivity in eating disorders. *Psychopharmacology Bulletin, 27,* 365–371.

MELZACK, R. (1986). Neurophysiological foundations of pain. In R. A. Sternbach (Ed.), *The psychology of pain* (2nd ed.). New York: Raven Press.

MISHARA, B. L., & KASTENBAUM, R. (1980). *Alcohol and old age.* New York: Grune & Stratton.

MOORCROFT, W. H. (1989). *Sleep, dreaming, and sleep disorders.* Lanham, MD: University Press of America.

MORRIS, G. O., WILLIAMS, H. L., & LUBIN, A. (1960). Misperception and disorientation during sleep deprivation. *Archives of General Psychiatry, 2,* 247–254.

NAPOLIELLO, M. J., & DOMANTAY, A. G. (1991). Buspirone: A worldwide update. *British Journal of Psychiatry, 159,* 40–44.

NOYES, R., CROWE, R. R., HARRIS, E. L., HAMRA, B. J., MCCHESNEY, C. M., & CHAUDHRY, D. R. (1986). Relationship between panic disorder and agoraphobia. *Archives of General Psychiatry, 43,* 227–232.

OKUMA, T. (1989). Acute and prophylactic properties of carbamazepine in bipolar affective disorders. In B. Lerer & S. Gershon (Eds.), *New directions in affective disorders* (pp. 535–539). New York: Springer-Verlag.

OLIN, B. R., HEBEL, S. K., DOMBEK, C. E., & KASTRUP, E. K. (Eds.). (1993). *Facts and comparison.* New York: Lippincott.

PARKES, J. D. (1985). *Sleep and its disorders.* Philadelphia: Saunders.

PELHAM, W. E. (1993). Pharmacotherapy with children with attention-deficit hyperactivity disorder. *School Psychology Review, 22,* 199–227.

PLOTKIN, D. A., GERSON, S. C., & JARVIK, L. F. (1987). Antidepressant drug treatment in the elderly. In H. Meltzer (Ed.), *Psychopharmacology: The third generation of progress* (pp. 1149–1158). New York: Raven Press.

PONTEROTTO, J. G. (1985). A counselor's guide to psychopharmacology. *Journal of Counseling and Development, 64*, 109–115.

PRICE, R. H., & LYNN, S. J. (1986). *Abnormal psychology* (2nd ed.). Pacific Grove, CA: Brooks/Cole.

REIMHERR, F. W., CHOUINARD, G., COHN, K., COLE, J., ITIL, T., LAPIERRE, Y., MASCO, H., & MENDELS, J. (1990). Antidepressant efficacy of sertraline: A double-blind, placebo- and amitriptyline-controlled, multicenter comparison study of outpatients with major depression. *Journal of Clinical Psychiatry, 51*, 18–27.

RESTAK, R. M. (1988). *The mind.* New York: Bantam Books.

RILEY, T. L. (1985). Normal sleep patterns. In T. E. Riley (Ed.), *Clinical aspects of sleep and sleep disturbance.* Boston: Butterworth.

ROSENBAUM, J. F. (1988). The course and treatment of manic-depressive illness: An update. *Journal of Clinical Psychiatry, 49*(11), 3–6.

ROY-BYRNE, P. P. (1992). Integrated treatment of panic disorder. *American Journal of Medicine, 92*(Suppl.), 49S–54S.

SANDERSON, W. C., & WETZLER, S. (1993). Observations on the cognitive behavioral treatment of panic disorder: Impact of benzodiazepines. *Psychotherapy, 30*, 125–132.

SCHATZBERG, A. F., & COLE, J. O. (1986). *Manual of clinical psychopharmacology.* Washington, DC: American Psychiatric Press.

SHUKLA, A., & COOK, B. L. (1989). Efficacy and safety of lithium-carbamazepine combination in mania. In B. Lerer & S. Gershon (Eds.), *New directions in affective disorders* (pp. 557–562). New York: Springer-Verlag.

SILVERSTONE, T. (1989). Psychopharmacology of schizoaffective mania. In B. Lerer & S. Gershon (Eds.), *New directions in affective disorders* (pp. 495–500). New York: Springer-Verlag.

SIRIS, S. G., BERMANZOHN, P., GONZALEZ, A., MASON, S., WHITE, C., & SHUWALL, M. (1991). The use of antidepressants for negative symptoms in a subset of schizophrenic patients. *Psychopharmacology Bulletin, 27*, 331–335.

SPENCER, E. K., KAFANTARIS, V., PADRON-GAYOL, M. V., ROSENBERG, C. R., & CAMPBELL, M. (1992). Haloperidol in schizophrenic children: Early findings from a study in progress. *Psychopharmacology Bulletin, 28*(2), 183–186.

STAHL, S. M. (1992). The current impact of neuroscience on psychotropic drug discovery and development. *Psychopharmacology Bulletin, 28*(1), 3–9.

STEWART, J. W., QUITKIN, F., & KLEIN, D. (1992). The pharmacotherapy of minor depression. *American Journal of Psychotherapy, 96*, 23–37.

SUPERNAW, R. B. (1991a). Pharmacotherapeutic management of acute pain. *U.S. Pharmacist,* pp. H-1, 2, 4, 7, 11, 13, 14.

SUPERNAW, R. B. (1991b). Recurrent headache syndromes. *U.S. Pharmacist,* pp. 33, 34, 37, 38, 42, 47, 48, 50, 52, & 54.

SWONGER, A. K., & MATEJSKI, M. P. (1991). *Nursing pharmacology.* Philadelphia: Lippincott.

SZEINBACH, S. L., & SUMMERS, K. H. (1992, May). Improving pharmacotherapeutic outcomes in panic disorder. *Drug Topics,* pp. 1–10.

TATRO, D. S., OW-WING, S. D., & HUIE, D. L. (1986). Drug toxicology. In A. M. Pagliaro & L. A. Pagliaro (Eds.), *Pharmacologic aspects of nursing* (pp. 180–187). St. Louis: Mosby.

TAYLOR, R. L. (1990). *Distinguishing psychological from organic disorders.* New York: Springer.

TEST, M. A., BURKE, S. S., & WALLISCH, L. S. (1990). Gender differences of young adults with schizophrenic disorders in community care. *Schizophrenia Bulletin, 16*(2), 331–344.

THOMAS, C. L. (Ed.). (1985). *Taber's cyclopedic medical dictionary* (15th ed.). Philadelphia: Davis.

TRIMBLE, M. R. (1990). Worldwide use of clomipramine. *Journal of Clinical Psychiatry, 51*(8)(Suppl.), 51–54.

TYRER, P. J., & SEIVEWRIGHT, N. (1984). Identification and management of benzodiazepine dependence. *Postgraduate Medical Journal, 60*(2), 41–46.

WALLIS, C., & WILLWERTH, J. (1992, July 6). Schizophrenia: A new drug brings patients back to life. *Time*, pp. 53–60.

WATERMAN, G. S., & RYAN, N. D. (1993). Pharmacological treatment of depression and anxiety in children and adolescents. *School Psychology Review, 22*, 228–242.

WINCOR, M. Z. (1990, January). Sleep disorders. *U.S. Pharmacist, 90*(01), pp. 26, 28–32, 35, 36, 41, 42, 44.

WOOLF, D. S. (1983). CNS depressants. In G. Bennett, C. Vourakis, & D. S. Woolf (Eds.), *Substance abuse*. New York: Wiley.

YESAVAGE, J. A. (1992). Depression in the elderly. *Postgraduate Medicine, 91*, 255–261.

MEDICATIONS INDEX

Index

Announcing an exciting new program on CD-ROM for the Macintosh

Exploring Psychological Disorders, Version 3.0
by Douglas L. Chute, Drexel University, and Margaret E. Bliss, MacLaboratory, Inc.
Single-copy price: $80. Site-license price: $100 plus $20/CPU

Based on Chute's award-winning **MacLaboratory for Psychology** program, this interactive software for CD-ROM on the Macintosh allows you to view authentic video clips of interviews with clients, work through diagnostic criteria, and use DSM-IV decision trees to diagnose a variety of clinical cases. In addition, you can explore animations on difficult-to-grasp concepts and use multimedia features including an interactive glossary, text, graphics, and movies.

The interactive nature of this "living book" makes it far more powerful than traditional videos. Scan quickly and efficiently through the movies to select any specific part; play them backward to select specific behaviors to study and analyze. The CD offers:

- Interactive access to decision trees, a hypertext glossary, and diagnostic criteria
- Decision trees that begin with clinical features of the Axis I disorders and allow users to follow a series of questions to include or exclude various disorders by clicking on the "yes" or "no" button
- Individual criteria for all the mental disorders on Axis I and Axis II of the DSM-IV, the GAF scales, and the Severity of Psychological Stressors Scale for Adults and Children. Eleven of the disorders are given full multimedia treatment, and the complete DSM-IV is included.

Topics Included in the Software
What Is Abnormal? / How Does It Go Wrong? Animations Showing Normal and Abnormal Brains for Their Neuroanatomy, Metabolic Activity, etc. / Vincent Van Gogh / How Do We Know? Film Clips of Researchers in Their Labs / Obsessive-Compulsive Disorder — Diagnosis and Case / Panic Disorder / Anna O. — The Real Story / Depression / Bipolar Case in a Manic and Depressed State / Eating Disorder / Erectile Dysfunction / Alcohol Abuse / Animation on Drugs and the Brain / Personality Disorders — Goering, Charles Manson / Cognitive Impairment / The Insanity Defense — John Hinckley, Jr.

Requires System 7, color monitor, and CD-ROM drive for the Macintosh®, Performa®, or PowerPC®.
Also available: Exploring Psychological Disorders: Clinical Projects Manual by Douglas Chute and Margaret Bliss walks users through activities and explorations.

ORDER FORM

Yes! Please send me *Exploring Psychological Disorders, Version 3.0*
_____ Single copy (ISBN: 0-534-23179-9) @ $80.
_____ Site license for CD-ROM (ISBN: 0-534-23181-8) @ $100 plus $20/CPU =

Subtotal _____

(Residents of AL, AZ, CA, CO, CT, FL, GA, IL, IN, KS, KY, LA, MA, MD, MI, MN, MO, NC, NJ, NY, OH, PA, RI, SC, TN, TX, UT, VA, WA, WI must add appropriate sales tax)   Tax _____

Payment Options   Handling _____
_____ Purchase Order enclosed. Please bill me.
_____ Check or Money Order enclosed.   Total _____

_____ Charge my _____ VISA _____ MasterCard _____ American Express

Card Number _____ Expiration Date _____

Signature_____

Please ship to: (Billing and shipping address must be the same.)

Name_____

Department _____ School _____

Street Address _____

City _____ State_____ Zip+4_____

Office phone number (_____) _____

_____ PLEASE SEND ME A COMPLIMENTARY COPY OF **EXPLORING PSYCHOLOGICAL DISORDERS: CLINICAL PROJECTS MANUAL** (ISBN: 0-534-23180-2)

You can fax your response to us at 408-375-6414 or e-mail your order to: info@brookscole.com
or detach, fold, secure, and mail with payment.

SECURE WITH TAPE

FOLD HERE

BUSINESS REPLY MAIL
FIRST CLASS   PERMIT NO. 358   PACIFIC GROVE, CA

POSTAGE WILL BE PAID BY ADDRESSEE

ATTN: _____ MARKETING _____

Brooks/Cole Publishing Company
511 Forest Lodge Road
Pacific Grove, California 93950-9968

FOLD HERE

TO THE OWNER OF THIS BOOK:

We hope that you have found *Counselor's Resource on Psychiatric Medications* useful. So that this book can be improved in a future edition, would you take the time to complete this sheet and return it? Thank you.

School and address: ————————————————————————————

Department: ——————————————————————————————

Instructor's name: —————————————————————————————

1. What I like most about this book is: —————————————————

————————————————————————————————————

————————————————————————————————————

2. What I like least about this book is: ————————————————

————————————————————————————————————

————————————————————————————————————

3. My general reaction to this book is: —————————————————

————————————————————————————————————

4. The name of the course in which I used this book is: ————————

————————————————————————————————————

5. Were all of the chapters of the book assigned for you to read? ——————

   If not, which ones weren't? ——————————————————————

6. In the space below, or on a separate sheet of paper, please write specific suggestions for improving this book and anything else you'd care to share about your experience in using the book.

————————————————————————————————————

————————————————————————————————————

————————————————————————————————————

————————————————————————————————————

————————————————————————————————————

Optional:

Your name: _____ Date: _____

May Brooks/Cole quote you, either in promotion for *Counselor's Resource on Psychiatric Medications* or in future publishing ventures?

Yes: _____ No: _____

Sincerely,

George Buelow
Suzanne Hebert

Brooks/Cole is dedicated to publishing quality publications for education in the human services fields. If you are interested in learning more about our publications, please fill in your name and address and request our latest catalogue, using this prepaid mailer.

Name: _____

Street Address: _____

City, State, and Zip: _____

FOLD HERE

NO POSTAGE
NECESSARY
IF MAILED
IN THE
UNITED STATES

FOLD HERE